AF726449

DRUGS *of* ABUSE

A Perspective

DRUGS *of* ABUSE
A Perspective

Donald W. Pfaff • Sandra Sherman

The Rockefeller University, USA

World Scientific

NEW JERSEY • LONDON • SINGAPORE • BEIJING • SHANGHAI • HONG KONG • TAIPEI • CHENNAI • TOKYO

Published by

World Scientific Publishing Co. Pte. Ltd.
5 Toh Tuck Link, Singapore 596224
USA office: 27 Warren Street, Suite 401-402, Hackensack, NJ 07601
UK office: 57 Shelton Street, Covent Garden, London WC2H 9HE

British Library Cataloguing-in-Publication Data
A catalogue record for this book is available from the British Library.

DRUGS OF ABUSE
A Perspective

Copyright © 2026 by World Scientific Publishing Co. Pte. Ltd.

All rights reserved. This book, or parts thereof, may not be reproduced in any form or by any means, electronic or mechanical, including photocopying, recording or any information storage and retrieval system now known or to be invented, without written permission from the publisher.

For photocopying of material in this volume, please pay a copying fee through the Copyright Clearance Center, Inc., 222 Rosewood Drive, Danvers, MA 01923, USA. In this case permission to photocopy is not required from the publisher.

ISBN 978-981-98-3147-0 (hardcover)
ISBN 978-981-98-3148-7 (ebook for institutions)
ISBN 978-981-98-3149-4 (ebook for individuals)

For any available supplementary material, please visit
https://www.worldscientific.com/worldscibooks/10.1142/14829#t=suppl

Contents

Introduction

At the start of the COVID-19 pandemic in 2020, drug overdose deaths in the U.S. numbered ~70,000 annually.[1] By the end of the pandemic in 2023, they numbered over 110,000, a 50% increase in four years.[2] By modern epidemiological standards, this rate of increase is shocking. While the number had come down to ~80,000 in 2024, it was still more than it was when pandemic-fueled overdose deaths had begun to rise.[3] Moreover, the latest hard numbers are in addition to "softer" figures regarding individuals struggling with addiction, whose treatment costs more than $500 billion annually.[4] When you add the downstream costs from lost production and criminal enforcement, the figure jumps to $800 billion — a year. This is about 2.5 times the FY2025 budget of California. Over the 15 years of the Vietnam War, 58,000 Americans died, and the government spent about US$168 billion (US$1.3 trillion in today's dollars). So, in effect, the human cost of drug addiction is equivalent to fighting one Vietnam War every 6 or 7 months; the economic cost is equivalent to fighting about 8 or 9 years of

---

[1] National Center for Health Statistics, Drug overdose deaths, https://www.cdc.gov/nchs/hus/topics/drug-overdose-deaths.htm

[2] National Institute on Drug Abuse, Drug overdose facts and figures, https://nida.nih.gov/research-topics/trends-statistics/overdose-death-rates#Fig1

[3] National Center for Health Statistics, https://www.cdc.gov/nchs/pressroom/nchs_press_releases/2025/20250514.htm

[4] Nestler EJ. (2025) The biology of addiction. *Sci Signaling* **18**(872), eadq0031.

the war every single year. The figures seem unfathomable. Either they make you feel entirely helpless or convince you that this is a national tragedy that each of us must try to address.

In 2024, we chose the latter course. But we also wondered how we could usefully add to the conversation, in view of the continuing research on addiction, the multiplicity of treatment options, and the books and articles available. In writing *Drugs of Abuse: A Perspective*, we decided that while we had not performed recent, cutting-edge research or devised a new mode of treatment, we could offer readers a new perspective on the problem of drug abuse, i.e., a new way of thinking about it that would integrate the various elements of the problem. How did it start? How do drugs operate in the brain? How are treatment modalities changing, and how may advances in "neurotechnology" radically change them in the coming years? No one, so far as we know, has put all this information in one place, which would help readers to grasp an enormous problem that is deeply embedded in social history. We hope that if people can see beyond the grim, daunting statistics to understand how drugs work, and why drugs have remained (a) so appealing and (b) so hard to eradicate, we can help them make their own contributions to combating the problem.

Our approach to *Drugs of Abuse* is straightforward. First, we provide a comprehensive history of how four representative drugs (cocaine, opium, alcohol, and tobacco) became addictive. Initially, they all started out as medications; how they were transformed into substances of abuse is a fascinating study in risk-taking, desperation, greed, and ignorance. We then examine the neurobiology of an array of addictive drugs, some radical proposals for combating addiction, and finally, how current efforts to eliminate or mitigate addiction now substantially depart from the 12-step program pioneered by Alcoholics Anonymous and are still largely intact in the Minnesota Model. But this is just a Table of Contents.

Our ultimate purpose is to examine the psychological and moral issues that have inflected drug addiction from biblical times (Noah got drunk after the flood!) to the present, where many treatment modalities walk a fine line between regimenting every action an addict takes and encouraging them to take charge of their own recovery. Once you appreciate how these issues play out in practice, you can formulate your own position — and, potentially, your own course of action.

Section 1 Origin Stories: Drugs of Abuse

This chapter will consider the origin stories of four representative drugs of abuse: cocaine, opium, alcoholic beverages, and tobacco. Each of these is ancient — in the case of alcohol and tobacco, their use dates to Paleolithic times. They all started out as medicines, or even sacred substances through which restricted groups of users venerated local deities. But then their use evolved. They became recreational, more widely available, and finally addictive. How did this happen? What was it about these drugs — or, that is, their sensory appeal — that enabled this evolution? How did societal developments, from the Romantic movement to the Industrial Revolution, act as accelerants? We'll discuss these questions.

Of course, the four drugs that we cite are all natural, i.e., they are derived from plants. They are not, in that sense, like many others that are synthesized in a lab — and are nightmarishly modern. But what the drugs in this chapter demonstrate, and why we chose to examine their origins, is that society can lose control over how drugs are used. An intended use can segue into uses that are unintended before ways are found to stall (much less reverse) the process. This is true for drugs like ketamine, an anesthetic that quickly became a "party drug."

Yet because the drugs in this chapter were initially medicinal, do their stories have any bearing on drugs like fentanyl, which were *designed* to be addictive, even before society lost control and they *became* addictive? Yes, because these older drugs still demonstrate that the desire to get high is embedded in human nature. So, when we are dealing with designer drugs (as well as drugs that have simply escaped our control), we need to find a way to neutralize that desire — literally, to make people less motivated to seek them out. Penalizing suppliers is an insufficient remedy, since the persistent desire will encourage new, even more deeply underground sources. In another Section, we discuss the neurochemistry of why some drugs are addictive and how to counteract the desire for them.

Chapter 1 – Cocaine

While cocaine is a refined, relatively modern product, consumption of its natural antecedent goes back at least to the middle of the first century B.C.E, when the coca plant was already being cultivated by indigenous peoples in South America.[1] The leaf (mixed with shell ash or chalk to enhance its strength) was chewed to extract the juice, and archeologists have found contemporaneous pottery "portraying the characteristic cheek bulge of the coca chewer."[2] The plant was a stimulant and appetite suppressant, though chewing was inefficient compared to the inhalation of today's (much more toxic) cocaine. As one observer notes:

> There is a limit to the number of leaves that even the most determined user can chew. The physical restraints of leaf chewing restrict the amount of cocaine that can be introduced into the bloodstream, and that acts as a safeguard against toxicity.[3]

---

[1] Calatayud J & González Á. (2003). History of the development and evolution of local anesthesia since the coca leaf. *Anesthesiology* **98**(6), 1503–1508.

[2] Petersen RC. (1977) Cocaine: an overview. *Drug Enforc* **4**(9).

[3] Karch SB. (1999) Cocaine: history, use, abuse. *J R Soc Med* **92**(8), 393–397.

Presumably, there was more time to chew in the afterlife. Archaeologists have found indigenous mummies buried with supplies of coca leaf. Similarly, pots from early Chinese tombs reveal the use of cannabis.[4] In Spain, fossilized poppy capsules, around 4200 years old, were recovered from small baskets found in a burial cave in the province of Granada.[5] Such gestures suggest the drugs' importance, especially regarding those who could afford a well-provisioned burial.

Yet while coca-chewing goes back well over two millennia, its heyday coincided with the Incan Empire (fl. 12th to 15th centuries) in what is now Peru, Bolivia, and Colombia. During that period, the plant was carefully cultivated and accorded "religious significance."[6] Access was restricted to the privileged classes, which, on occasion, deigned to grant access to those beneath them as a sign of favor — for example, soldiers engaged in combat and workers engaged in one of the massive municipal projects still evident among the ruins. It was also used in the aftermath of successful military actions. As Peter Andreas observes, coca "facilitated" the Incas' pacification and co-optation of conquered tribal leaders, who were given bales of coca leaves once they pledged their loyalty. Conquered communities also paid tribute to the Incas with gold, silver, and coca.[7]

---

[4] Phelan M. (2019). Ancient pots from Chinese tombs reveal early use of cannabis. AAAS, https://www.aaas.org/news/ancient-pots-chinese-tombs-reveal-early-use-cannabis.

[5] Merlin MD. (2003) Archeological evidence for the tradition of psychoactive plant use in the old world. *Econ Bot* **57**, 295–323.

[6] Petersen.

[7] Andreas P. (2022) *Killer High: A History of War in Six Drugs*. Oxford University Press, 207.

But apart from chewing, did the drug have uses that foreshadowed cocaine's later medicalization? Evidence suggests that it was employed as an analgesic in crude trepanations, where the skull was opened to allow evil spirits to escape. While the patient's next stop may have been to be buried with the leaf, Petersen cites "evidence that the operation was sometimes a success in that the victim survived."

Of course, the Incan empire itself did not survive; as it declined, so did many of the restrictions surrounding coca. By the time of Francisco Pizzaro's 16th-century advance on Cuzco, the plant's religious and class-based connotations were largely gone. Most people could, if they wished, chew it habitually. Yet this very accessibility was what now appealed to the Spanish, who recognized that if local populations were to be subjugated under brutal conditions — for example, in silver and gold mining — then coca was necessary to keep them motivated. The Spanish even encouraged coca's cultivation, overcoming concerns that the plant's residual religious associations would impede the Incas' conversion.

At this point, coca's medicalization — and, hence, the first glimmerings of cocaine, also at first a medicine — began to emerge. The Spanish, who despite being Western and Christian, were no more "scientific" than the Incas, recognized that coca was a potent folk remedy for common problems ranging from stomach ailments to muscle aches, skin disorders, and toothaches.[8] In 1609, Padre Blas Valera wrote:

> Coca protects the body from any ailments, and our doctors use it in powdered form to reduce the swelling of wounds, to strengthen

---

[8] See Calatayud, n.1 supra, for an excellent discussion of the Spanish interest in coca.

> broken bones, and to expel cold from the body or prevent it from entering, and to cure rotten wounds or sores that are full of maggots. And if it does so much for outward aliments, will not its singular virtue have even greater effect in the entrails of those who eat it?[9]

The question posed by Valera suggests that coca might have pervasive internal effects, anticipating claims made for cocaine over two centuries later.

The first reference to coca's anesthetic effects appears in a mid-17th-century work by Spanish Jesuit Bernabe Cobo, who wrote that his toothache was relieved by chewing coca:

> [A] monk friend of mine… advised me to chew for a few days on *Coca*. As I did, indeed, soon to find my toothache gone.[10]

In the tradition of cocaine enthusiasts, including Karl Koller, Sigmund Freud, and William Halsted, Cobo tried the drug on himself.

Spanish enthusiasm grew to the extent that, in the mid-18th century, a former Jesuit recommended that coca be given to working people generally to enhance their health and productivity. As unreconstructed colonialists, the Spanish figured that if they could popularize the drug in Europe, they could corner the market with exports. Did they realize that seeking to restore coca's class-based connotations, which the Incas had largely abandoned, would be cruelly ironic? Apparently not. Another mid-18th-century student of the drug, Captain Antonio d'Alloa, remarked:

[9] Inter-Andean Institute of Coca Sciences, The precious leaf called coca, https://web.archive.org/web/20161230070400/https://cienciadelacoca.org/CocaVega.html

[10] Cobo, B. (1653) *Historia del Neuvo Mundo*. Vol. I, Book 5, Chapter xxix.

> This herb is so nutritious and invigorating that the Indians labor whole days without anything else, and on the want of it they find decay in their strength.[11]

Some 18th-century social engineers were tantalized by the idea of maintaining workers' productivity while offering them minimal nourishment. In Great Britain, for example, Count Rumford, Sir Frederick Eden, and several others contrived diets for the poor based on the minimal caloric intake required to produce an expected quantum of work.[12] So, coca should have had a major impact. But it didn't.

The drug failed to catch on in Europe because the leaves deteriorated over the long sea voyage and, as the Europeans quickly learned, the plant could not grow in the cold European climate. Moreover, there was at least one warning about the negative effects of abusing coca. After a voyage to the Amazon (1827–1832), the German doctor and naturalist Eduard Poeppig described an array of symptoms, including weakness, headaches, personality changes, and weight loss, that accompanied coca consumption, and observed that coca consumers were unable to kick their habit. They were, he said, considered beneath alcoholics.

Nonetheless, by the mid-19th century, the tide was beginning to turn. In his monograph, *Plant Intoxicants* (1855), the explorer and biochemist Baron Ernst von Bibra disagreed with Poeppig, observing that during his own visit to South America, he witnessed the positive, energizing effects of coca on the indigenous population. Its effects on himself were modest. But Italian neurologist Paolo Mantegazza was full of praise for the plant. His 1859 monograph, *On the Hygienic and Medical Values of Coca*, based

---

[11] Cited in Petersen.

[12] Sherman S. (2001) *Imagining Poverty: Quantification and the Decline of Paternalism.* Ohio State University Press.

on personal experimentation, found that coca induced an altered mental state characterized by phantasmagoric, kaleidoscopic images. Coca raised his pulse rate. He became euphoric. In other words, he shifted from von Bibra's workaday concerns toward what we might call a "psychedelic" experience. Later in life, he took cocaine enthusiastically.

The arc of Mantegazza's personal history parallels the transformation of coca — a natural substance — into cocaine.

It took until well into the 19th century for cocaine to be refined from coca; by then, it was cocaine and not coca leaves that drew significant interest. Cocaine was in use extensively by the 1880s. The great fictional detective, Sherlock Holmes, was an avid user. In *The Sign of Four* (1890), Holmes' friend and assistant, Dr. Watson, offers a graphic description of Holmes' injecting himself with the famous "seven percent solution" of the drug. The first synthesis and description of the cocaine molecule occurred in 1898, though subsequent efforts continued to make refinements.[13] The suffix "-caine" referred to the substance's ability to act as a local anesthetic (think of Novocain).

Cocaine became respectable, morphing from a dystopian means to extract work from the poor to a drug that diminished pain. In a famous experiment of 1884, a close associate of Sigmund Freud, Karl Koller, applied cocaine in solution to his own eye and then pricked it with pins. He presented his findings to the Heidelberg Ophthalmologic Society. Around the same time, cocaine was demonstrated to be useful as a nerve-blocker and in peridural and spinal anesthesia.[14]

---

[13] Total synthesis of cocaine (Willstatter), https://total-synthesis.com/cocaine-synthesis/

[14] On cocaine's anesthetic applications, see Kayser O. (2024) *From the Maluku to Molecules: How Natural Substances Write History*. Springer, 37–69.

Freud

But the medicalization of cocaine had serious "side effects." In 1884, Freud encouraged one of his patients, Ernst von Fleischl, to break his morphine addiction by taking cocaine — von Fleischl instead became one of the earliest cocaine addicts. *That* addiction was far worse than his addiction to morphine, but Freud was too late in realizing his mistake and in withdrawing Fleischl's supply of the drug. To be fair, Freud may have been following the current practice of treating morphine addiction with cocaine. But Freud was nonetheless under a serious misimpression concerning cocaine based on his own experimentation with the drug. In *Uber Coca* (1884), he wrote that cocaine induces:

> Exhilaration and lasting euphoria, which in no way differs from the normal euphoria of the healthy person. You perceive an increase of self-control and possess more vitality and capacity for work. In other words, you are simply normal, and it is soon hard to believe you are under the influence of any drug.[15] Long intensive physical work is performed without any physical fatigue. This result is enjoyed without any of the unpleasant after-effects that follow exhilaration brought about by alcoholic beverages.
>
> No craving for the further use of cocaine appears after the first, or even after repeated taking of the drug.

[15] There is a striking similarity between Freud's claim of feeling "normal" when taking cocaine and that of Thomas De Quincey in *Confessions of an Opium-eater* (1821), where he asserts that opium just made him feel like himself. Of course, De Quincey later went on to relate his astonishing, surrealistic dreams while under the influence — an experience that Freud would have recognized.

Freud specifically, perhaps fatally, praises Mantegazza as an influence.

It is well-known that Freud and his contemporary, the brilliant father of modern surgery, William Halsted, became cocaine addicts. As a result, Freud developed chest pain and became depressed. His nose was so congested that he had to have it surgically opened. It is said that the "Model Dream" in his famous *Interpretation of Dreams* (1895) was induced by cocaine. He remained addicted for 15 years, and only quit when he almost killed his patient Emma Eckstein, ironically by cauterizing her nose with cocaine.[16] Halsted, who practiced and taught at Johns Hopkins, essentially withdrew from medicine. He committed himself to an insane asylum. But he never fully recovered. He had fallen into addiction because, like many physicians of the period, he experimented on himself, injecting himself with cocaine to determine its numbing effect in place of general anesthesia.[17]

Freud and Halsted were the leading edge of cocaine's massive casualty list. Calatayud observes:

> After Koller's discovery of cocaine's local anesthetic powers, its use spread rapidly, but because it was administered in high

---

[16] Cohen D. (2011). *Freud on Coke*. Andrews UK Limited.

[17] Self-experimentation with drugs was a common practice during the 19th century. As Mike Jay observes, it had "well-recognized protocols and reporting conventions. In an age of experiment, when scientific and medical breakthroughs often involved personal risk, sampling an unknown drug was seen as no more reckless than the anatomical experiments, electric shocks, or toxic exposure to which the researchers of the day routinely subjected themselves." In fact, "the writings of these self-experimenters were a source of intense fascination to the wider public." Jay M. (2023) *Psychonauts: Drugs and the Making of the Modern Mind*. Yale University Press, 6–7, 8.

concentrations (on the order of 10 to 30%), practitioners soon began to report its alarming side effects. Between 1884 and 1891, 200 cases of systemic intoxication and 13 deaths attributed to the drug were recorded, quenching enthusiasm for it and prompting physicians to turn to gases such as nitrous oxide in dentistry. Furthermore, about this time, the addictive effects of cocaine began to emerge as several early users, Freud and Halsted among them, fell victim to it.

But if Freud and Halsted were chastened, and physicians were moved to seek safer alternatives, the 19th century still boomed with coca/cocaine comestibles. In 1863, French chemist Angelo Mariani started selling Vin Mariani, a Bordeaux treated with coca leaves. The ethanol in the wine served to extract cocaine from the leaves, and Pope Leo XIII gave Mariani a medal. Ultimately, Mariani published 13 volumes of testimonials from figures such as Henrik Ibsen, Sarah Bernhardt, the Prince of Wales, H. G. Wells, and Thomas Edison. In 1885, the American pharmaceutical maker, Parke-Davis, mass-marketed coca-leaf cigarettes, a cocaine inhalant, and related cocaine products that it claimed could eliminate pain.[18] It claimed that "an enumeration of the diseases in which coca and cocaine have been found of serious service would include a category of almost all the maladies that flesh is heir to."[19] Freud was an initial customer.

There were, in fact, an array of patent medicine manufacturers who, in the days before drug regulation, sold coca- and cocaine-laced products, including ointments, throat lozenges, suppositories, nose powders, and sprays. Petersen states that "they allegedly

[18] Musto DF. (1989) America's first cocaine epidemic. *Wilson Q.* **13**(3), 59–64.
[19] Cited in Musto, supra.

cured an equally wide range of disorders, including alcoholism, asthma, colds, corns, eczema, neuralgia, opiate addiction, and venereal disease." Contemporary Sears, Roebuck catalogs made these remedies easy to get, no matter where one lived. A vast number of people consumed cocaine for a vast array of reasons.

Yet when it came to black people, the story was different. Recently emancipated black men often had back-breaking jobs on the docks, railways, and as porters. They might have relied on cocaine to enhance their endurance. But racist journalism claimed that cocaine weakened their morals and could make them temporarily insane. Of course, the subtext was that white women were endangered, perpetuating a stereotype of black men that was shaped by the slave economy. Well into the 20th century, in fact, Jim Crow associations between blacks and cocaine-driven behavior still found outlets. In 1914, the *New York Times* featured a headline blaring "Negro cocaine 'fiends' are a new Southern menace."[20] In his 1931 song, "Minnie the Moocher," Cab Calloway described Smokey Joe as "cokey."

It was the South that also gave the world Coca-Cola. Everyone knows that the original recipe for Coca-Cola (1886), formulated in Atlanta, contained an extract of the coca leaf — cocaine. But in 1903, in response to rising concerns about the drug, Coca-Cola became cocaine-free (while keeping coca in its name). But what most people don't know is that Coke was originally advertised as a patent medicine, "a valuable BRAIN tonic and cure for all nervous affections." Judging from current TV commercials, Coke may still be making some of the same insinuations.

---

[20] An image of the headline, and accompanying story, appears in Fisher CE. (2022) *The Urge: Our History of Addiction*. Penguin, 131.

Chapter 2 – Opium

The preserved remains of opium seeds were discovered in a 7000-year-old Neolithic city submerged in an Italian lake northwest of Rome. M.D. Merlin observed that the seeds were "presumably cultivated for food, oil, medicine, and possibly cult use."[21] The discovery, which has all the mythic connotations of finding a submerged Atlantis, is even more suggestive because the remains were near a "Great Mother" votive figure — apparently, the seeds *were* involved with a cult. As in the case of coca, opium's medicinal and psychoactive properties found an outlet in religious expression. Might they even have been the basis for it? These old remains make us reflect on the role of drugs in cultural development, long before such drugs began to be abused.

Archeological remains in other places around the Mediterranean indicate medicinal and spiritual uses for the opium poppy. Seeds were discovered in the cellar of an ancient Roman farmhouse near Pompeii, situated to suggest that they were part of a "medicinal preparation"; there was also a "poppy seed cake" in Pompeii, probably honoring the goddess Isis/Demeter.[22] Seeds were found near a Spanish burial site, which were laid down 4200 years ago.[23] In the National Museum of Antiquities, Cyprus, there is a vase dating

---

[21] Merlin, supra, at n. 5.

[22] Merlin, citing Ciaraldi M. (2000) Drug preparation in evidence: An unusual plant and bone assemblage from the Pompeiian countryside, Italy. *Veg Hist Archaeobot* **9**, 91, and Ciaraldi M & Richardson J. (2000) Food, ritual, and rubbish in the making of Pompeii. *Proceedings of the Ninth Annual Theoretical Roman Archaeology Conference*. Oxbow Books.

[23] Merlin. See also Inglis L. (2019). *Milk of Paradise: A History of Opium.* Pegasus Books, p. 6, citing a Neolithic burial site near Barcelona, Spain, where a man

from the second millennium B.C.E. that was apparently used to inhale opium vapor, and that was found in a cult chamber on Crete. A terracotta goddess from Crete with "uplifted hands and a trance-like facial expression" was found together with paraphernalia that indicate probable inhalation of opium vapors."[24]

The goddess embodies, so to speak, the connection between religion and the power of opium to induce hallucination. In this regard, one scholar suggests that the goddess could also represent a "priestess hallucinating for the purpose of uttering prophecies."[25] Opium enabled her to connect the mundane and the divine — the drug was not just some inert offering to a distant god. Its power (at least insofar as it was recognized in culture) was to induce transcendence; coca's power was mundane, enabling workers to work longer.

Similar archeological evidence for opium use, including a ritualistic pipe, was found around Cyprus.[26] In fact, the island was central to an extensive trade network that during the late second millennium B.C.E., supplied the Eastern Mediterranean with opium for medicinal and ritualistic purposes. So, it is not surprising that artifacts of opium use have been found in much of the

---

was interred with "a poppy seed capsule stuck in his bad teeth and his bones contained evidence of long-term opium consumption."

[24] Merlin, citing Kritikos PG & Papadaki SP. (1967) The history of the poppy and opium and their expansion in antiquity in the eastern Mediterranean area. *Bull Narc* **19**, 3.

[25] Merrillees RS. (1962) Opium trade in the Bronze Age Levant. *Antiquity* **36**, 287–192.

[26] While smoking was one means of consuming opium, it could also be ingested, applied to the skin, and even absorbed through anal suppositories. Mixed with hemlock, it offered a painless way to commit suicide (or to be executed).

Middle East.[27] They have also been found in Greece, where the ancient culture "associated fertility and abundance with the opium poppy."[28] As reflections of its cultural and economic importance during the period, images of the opium poppy appear on contemporary Greek, Roman, and even Jewish coins. Whatever its transcendental connotations, opium was commodified (and in this sense was a fitting image to be stamped on coins).

Nor was the opium trade just around the Mediterranean. Radiocarbon and stratigraphic dating of archeological remains demonstrates that as far back as 3000 B.C.E., opium was used all over Europe (including what is now the United Kingdom [U.K.]). There is evidence for its use in Medieval Germany. The Vikings cultivated it north of Denmark, based on evidence from the 11th century.[29] It is embedded in Europe's cultural inheritance, and is not some "exotic" substance that found its way into Europe (the way coca did) by way of early modern colonialism. Opium was around in Europe for millennia before Columbus. In fact, when he sailed to the New World, he was briefed to bring opium back.[30]

But in the first millennium, as the Roman Empire ceased to dominate the Mediterranean, Arabs moved into the opium trade. They introduced the drug to China and India. Islamic physicians used the drug as an anesthetic. Later, it was used to treat migraines

---

[27] Egyptian medical texts from the second century B.C.E. feature opium. See, for example, *The Therapeutic Papyrus of Thebes*, dated 1552 B.C.E.

[28] Merlin.

[29] Inglis, supra, at 46.

[30] Booth M. (2013) *Opium: A History*. St. Martin's Griffin, p. 22. Booth indicates that other early explorers — Cabot, Magellan, Vasco da Gama — were all required to find opium.

as well as an array of maladies, including sexual dysfunction.[31] What's interesting, however, is that in the Islamic world — where intoxicants were prohibited — opium lost its ritualistic, psychoactive importance and was treated as purely medicinal.

By the time of the drug's popularization in Europe in the 16th and 17th centuries (where it was a contemporary of coca), it was being recommended for pain and insomnia.[32] It was a remedy for dysentery, cholera, and diarrhea based on its proclivity for hardening stool (this could, of course, lead to constipation, a chronic affliction of those who were addicted). During the 18th century, it was used to treat nervous disorders, though withdrawal could lead to serious depression.[33] At this point, its most common means of consumption was as laudanum, a tincture of powdered opium (10% by weight) in alcohol that became a semi-respectable means of addiction. It was listed in the *London Pharmacopeia* (1618). In *Genera Plantarum* (1753), it was first classified by Linnaeus.[34]

In 18th-century England, opium was the subject of a fierce battle. In 1753, for example, George Young's *A Treatise on Opium* sought to counter medical praise for the substance, arguing that "opium is a poison by which great numbers are daily destroyed." But opium, and its derivative morphine, remained in use, particularly

[31] See Avicenna's *Canon of Medicine*, completed in 1025. The text was extremely influential.

[32] See, for example, Sydenham T. (1676) *Medical Observations*.

[33] Kramer JC. (1979) Opium rampant: Medical use, misuse and abuse in Britain and the West in the 17th and 18th centuries. *Br J Addict Alcohol Other Drugs*, **74**(4), 377–389.

[34] Martin Booth observes that Linnaeus, "like many of his contemporaries, and generations before him, he was well aware of [opium's] capabilities." See Booth, 1.

when mixed with other ingredients — for example, brandy, whiskey, and belladonna. It was used in surgery, even as patients were tied down and restrained.[35] Research into Eighteenth Century Collections Online, a searchable database that includes every known written work during the period, identifies 12,320 separate works that mention "opium." Here is an example from Edward Ward's *London Spy* (1700), which pits the author's own brand of medication against substances (including opium) that can kill you:

> It is absolutely Necessary for all Persons to carry in their Pockets, for who knows how the Passions of Love, Fear, Anger, Despair, Jealousie, or the like, by the subtle insinuations of Satan, who is watchful of all opportunities, may prevail upon you, to offer violence to your most pretious [sic] Lives, by taking Rats-bane, Mercury, Arsnick, and the like. (7).

The 18th century *knew* about the dangers of opium,[36] even if addiction had not yet been scientifically identified as a chronic brain disease.[37] In his *Metaphysics of Morals* (1797), Immanuel Kant warned that opium produces a "dreamy euphoria" that could make one "silent, reticent, and withdrawn."

---

[35] Adkins L & Adkins R. (2013) *Eavesdropping on Jane Austen's England: How Our Ancestors Lived Two Centuries Ago*. Hachette UK.

[36] Knowledge of opium's effects was hardly new; it was already available in the 17th century. See, for example, Richard Short, *Of Drinking Water, Against Our Novelists, that Prescribe it in England* (1656), which denigrates consuming the local water on grounds that "we may as well give Narcoticks, that is, stupefying things, as poppy, and opium."

[37] On the history of how addiction has been defined and studied, see Fisher, supra, at n. 18. In *Mysteries of Opium Reveal'd* (1700), Dr. John Jones provides a vivid description of addiction, probably based on his own experience.

Still, by the 19th century, laudanum was in a vast array of patent medicines, such as Godfrey's Cordial and Mother Bailey's Quieting Syrup. It was given to women for menstrual cramps and vague "feminine complaints." It was given to children. It was used to treat symptoms of cholera and yellow fever that tore through Britain's cramped cities before the adoption of public sanitation. Doctors resisted focusing on their remedies' potential to cause addiction. It was not until later in the century that serious attention to addiction, as a disease, began to take hold; it was mostly prompted by the effects of morphine, opium's much more potent derivative.

In the United States (U.S.), opium pills and opiates (such as laudanum and morphine) were used in massive amounts to relieve pain and suffering among soldiers during the Civil War. As a result, countless veterans became addicted, dubbing their addiction "opium slavery" and "morphine mania."[38] President Lincoln's wife, Mary, was a laudanum addict. Opium was a constituent of American patent medicines until, by the 20th century, regulation began to limit its use.

---

[38] See Virginia Museum of History and Culture, Opium addiction in the Civil War's aftermath, https://virginiahistory.org/learn/opiate-addiction-civil-wars-aftermath#:~:text=Countless%20veterans%20became%20addicted%20to,severe%20consequences%20for%20veterans'%20lives. On the stigmatization of addicted veterans as immoral and unmanly, see Jones JS. (2020) Opium slavery: Civil War veterans and opium addiction. *J Civ War Era* **10**:2, 185–212. Doctors were largely blamed for causing the addiction because of over-prescription, and, after the war, ex-military surgeons urged that opioids be prescribed sparingly. See Jones JS. (2025) *Opium Slavery: Civil War Veterans and America's First Opioid Crisis*. University of North Carolina Press.

Yet as the soldiers' addiction portended, it was morphine that became the most acute problem. Morphine could be delivered by the newly invented hypodermic syringe, which came to the U.S. from Britain in the 1850s. Physicians could administer precise quantities of the drug, which, in medical circles, gained a "scientific" patina. But anyone who could obtain a syringe could inject themselves, and morphine use (and abuse) spread rapidly — in the U.S. and abroad. In 1870, doctors began to react: a small group met at the New York City YMCA to establish the American Association for the Cure of Inebriates. The idea was that problems with drugs and alcohol were *medical* problems and should be treated like any other disease. It was a stunning, ironic turnaround, since so many doctors had initially prescribed morphine with few inhibitions.

But the problem wasn't just medical. Could medical treatment compete with the sheer desire to get high?

The rationale for recreational drug-taking was available in 19th-century literature, which had given addiction an aesthetic appeal. In Thomas De Quincey's *Confessions of an Opium-Eater* (1821), which is the locus classicus of that literature, the opium dreams that take up much of Book II are gorgeous, riveting even, two centuries later, when we are accustomed to psychedelic art. They might almost be read to justify the withdrawal symptoms that De Quincey also describes (the ratio of gorgeous to harrowing is unmistakably tipped toward the former). There is a reason why many of the Romantic poets — among them Samuel Taylor Coleridge, Percy Bysshe Shelley, John Keats, and Lord Byron — are associated with opium. Unlike cocaine, opium is woven into the Western imagination. If it is a soporific and painkiller (and in pre-scientific times, a panacea), it is also, literally, the stuff of dreams.

In fact, *Confessions* was a runaway bestseller and was widely translated. In France, for example, Baudelaire translated parts of it in *Les Paradis Artificiels* (1860).[39] *Confessions* created the archetype of the drug addict and offered readers the first compelling narrative of opium's power to seduce.[40] Predictably, *The Family Oracle of Health* (1824) condemned it for causing misery and for leading to abuse. But no matter. Salvador Dali, Jean Cocteau, and Pablo Picasso — all admitted users — are De Quincey's direct descendants.

Yet in many staggeringly important respects, and despite centuries of opium use in the West, no history of opium is complete without examining its role in Chinese history. Opium was known in China since the 15th century and was touted for its ability to prolong sex. It was consumed in polite society, where it was smoked by cognoscenti in a languorous ritual along with taking tea. The experience is captured in this contemporary account:

> On a miserable rainy day, when you feel down, light up an opium lamp on a low table, recline face to face, pass the pipe around and inhale. At first there is a sudden feeling of refreshment, one's head and eyes becoming very clear. Soon afterwards, there is quietude and profound well-being. After a while, one's bones and joints become extremely relaxed and the eyes heavy. This is followed

---

[39] M. Jay, supra, states that when the translation appeared, it "would become a ubiquitous reference point for the fevered drug culture of the *fin-de-siecle*," 51.
[40] Fisher, supra at n. 29, calls *Confessions* a "landmark... the first literary text devoted to drug use and the first addiction memoir." It is, moreover, a "celebration of opium, a love letter, a polemic, even a religious text," 100. Yest because De Quincey never really kicked the habit, Fisher also calls *Confessions* "a highbrow fable that masked a devastating reality," 106.

> by a gradual descent into slumber, and detached from all worries, one enters a world of dreams and fantasies, completely free like a spirit.[41]

Like fine carpets, music boxes, and watches, opium consumption became another marker of urban, civilized — hedonistic — life. Caquet notes that rich families employed opium butlers. They acquired the finest paraphernalia as opium became "part of Chinese hospitality, male companionship, and celebratory rituals."[42]

By the 18th century, opium was smoked by a large portion of the population in a tobacco mixture called madak. Eighteenth and early 19th-century Chinese emigrants to cities such as San Francisco, London, and New York brought the opium habit with them. The magnificent TV series *Warrior* (2019–2023), produced by Bruce Lee, dramatizes San Francisco's underworld of opium commerce and the related tong wars among rival Chinese factions. It also depicts further battles, which pitted nativists (including Irish immigrants, who fought for the North in the Civil War) against the Chinese. The conflict, where the Americans attacked the Chinese for corrupting their culture, ultimately led to the Chinese Exclusion Act of 1882.

China first attempted to ban opium in 1729, but the ban only reached sellers; users were exempt. A full-scale ban was adopted in 1799 with various crackdowns that continued through 1860. For example, in 1813, the emperor issued a major decree against it, apparently prompted by his discovery that his son and heir had dabbled in the drug (there was damning evidence in a set of verses by the prince). In fact, as Caquet observes, it was in China, not the

[41] Cited in Caquet PE. (2022) *Opium's Orphans: The 200-Year History of the War on Drugs*. Reaktion Books, at 20.
[42] Caquet, 28.

West, where modern attempts to limit opium consumption originated.[43] But perhaps because the ban created so much obvious danger for those who risked punishment by flouting it, smugglers could raise their prices. The effect, ironically, was that smuggling gained increasing appeal, and larger amounts of opium began entering the country. Ultimately, however, increasing supplies, stoked by the British East India Company, caused prices to fall.

The Chinese debated whether legalizing opium might reduce its appeal as well as the will to engage in smuggling. The debate sounds very 21st century. But in the end, the prohibitions were hardened and began to bite British merchants who were brazenly selling into the Chinese market. In fact, the Chinese dumped tons of opium into the sea (while apologizing to the sea for causing pollution).

At the same time, the British were concerned for their trade balance with China, since while British citizens fancied Chinese tea, cotton, and furniture, the Chinese were uninterested in British goods. To rectify the imbalance, the British began smuggling opium (which had always entered China through British India and was also a prop to its economy). When the Chinese took action to halt the smuggling, the British commenced the first Opium War in 1839. The British won, taking Hong Kong and winning, as well, several major concessions (but still not the legalization of opium). Other foreign powers, including the U.S., also won concessions.[44]

---

[43] Caquet, supra.

[44] Though Britain dominated the opium trade with China, the U.S. was no bystander. As Andreas observes, "[M]ost of the U.S. firms that began conducting trade in China had trafficked in opium in the years leading up to the outbreak of war. Warren Delano II, the grandfather of Franklin Delano Roosevelt and the creator of the family fortune, profited from shipping opium to China . . ." *Killer High*, 147–148.

The war sparked fierce opposition, with claims that the opium trade was immoral. Yet the trade continued. China was defeated again in the Second Opium War (1857–1858), making further concessions to the West and finally legalizing opium imports. But in reaction, it began to produce opium on a massive scale. This domestic product eventually became cheaper than imported opium, and even the lowest classes had access to it. Rickshaw pullers took it to soothe their muscles. Among women, foot-binding was still a common practice, and opium eased the pain.

Of course, despite the drug's accessibility, not everyone who smoked opium was an addict. But addiction spread across all classes. In 1837, the *Chinese Repository* described a series of paintings by a Chinese artist illustrating a smoker's descent from "health and wealth to pain and poverty."[45] The poor had opium dens, where they often stupefied themselves in filthy conditions.

In the 19th century, remorseful missionary societies sought to combat the spread of opium in China, but it was not until the early 20th century that the Chinese again took the initiative, publicly burning opium paraphernalia and acting against opium farmers. Smokers had to be licensed, and their rations were gradually reduced. Yet the campaign was only marginally successful, and some food-growing areas were cleared for increased opium poppy production. It took a ruthless crackdown by the Chinese Communists to finally eliminate production and consumption, even though it appears that opium was crucial to Party finances as it came into power. Production shifted to Southeast Asia, where some American soldiers picked up the habit in Vietnam.

---

[45] Booth, 89.

Chapter 3 – Alcoholic Beverages

This section examines the history of three distinct types of beverages — beer, wine, and distilled spirits — that have been consumed over the millennia. Each has its own history, though their development reflects many similar motivations (e.g., the need to retard spoilage of their constituent ingredients), and the development of beer often intertwines with that of wine.

Beer

The term "beer" often refers to fermented grain-based beverages, hopped or not. But technically, only by adding hops is beer "beer." Because in practice, this distinction rarely matters, we have not limited our discussion to what is technically "beer." Instead, we follow Franz Muessdoerffer's approach in "A comprehensive history of beer brewing," where he concludes that while he cannot cover all grain-based fermented beverages, "a consideration of hopped beer only would be too selective and would ignore the fundamental roots of brewing technology and beer culture."[46] Besides, these roots are fascinating.

Archaeologists speculate that beer-making was more fundamental to the development of sedentary agriculture (around 10,000 B.C.E.) than was the cultivation of grain for bread.[47]

---

[46] Meussdoerffer FG. (2009) A comprehensive history of beer brewing, in *Handbook of Brewing: Processes, Technology, Markets.* Wiley-VCH Verlag GmbH & Co., 1–42, at 1.

[47] Andreas, supra, at 16, citing Wadley G & Hayden B. (2015) Pharmacologic influences on the neolithic transition. *J Ethnobiol* **35**:3, 566–584; Liu L, *et al.* (2018) Fermented beverage and food storage in 13,000 y-old stone mortars at

In any case, the yeast in beer (and its related fermented grain product, ale), for much of history, was fundamental to the process of *baking* bread. For example, in Hannah Glasse's mid-18th-century blockbuster, *The Art of Cookery Made Plain and Easy*, the recipe for French Bread instructs the baker to add "a Pint and a half of good Ale-yeast" to the flour mixture as leaven. Conveniently, this recipe is preceded by an extensive discussion of Rules for Brewing, since a well-functioning kitchen needed a supply of the yeast that rose to the top of the ale and could be scooped off. Until packaged yeast was invented in the 19th century, fermenting grain was the source of leavening,[48] and most baked products — even sweet ones — had a slightly fermented tang. Teetotalers (if there were any) would still have been intimate with beer, if only indirectly.

Beer goes way back in human history. If we have always consumed it to get a buzz, archaeologists who study fermented beverages (this includes wine as well as beer) offer a more comprehensive rationale. The "intensification of agriculture" is part of it, but it goes much further:

> This nearly universal phenomenon of fermented beverage production is explained by ethanol's combined analgesic, disinfectant, and profound mind-altering effects. Moreover, fermentation helps to

---

Raqefet Cave, Israel: Investigating Natufian Ritual Feasting. *J Arch Sci Rep* **21**, 783–793, and citations therein. Liu concludes by stating: "Beer brewing may have been, at least in part, an underlying motivation to cultivate cereal in the Southern Levant, supporting the hypothesis proposed more than 60 years ago," 792.

[48] It was possible to make sourdough leavening using dough from the previous batch, but *that* batch (or the batch before it) was, of course, originally made with ale-yeast (also called "barm").

> preserve and enhance the nutritional value of foods and beverages. Because of their perceived pharmacological, nutritional, and sensory benefits, fermented beverages thus have played key roles in the development of human culture and technology, contributing to the advance and intensification of agriculture, horticulture, and food-processing techniques. Among all strata of society, they have marked major life events, from birth to death, as well as victories, auspicious events, and harvests, etc.[49]

As this passage suggests, beer production is in some respects analogous to cheese-making: in the long eons before refrigeration, grain (and milk) could be preserved through fermentation.[50] Their nutritional value could be "enhanced" because just as aged cheese is easier to digest than milk (e.g., for the lactose intolerant),[51] beer is easier to eat and digest because you don't expend as much energy chewing raw grain; you don't have to break down the complex carbohydrates with the ptyalin in saliva, and you don't even have to spend time cooking the grain down into gruel. Finally, the passage mentions the "sensory benefits" of fermentation, that is, fermented products taste good; their taste can also vary — beer, like

---

[49] McGovern P, Zhang J, Tang J, *et al.* (2004) Fermented beverages of pre- and proto-historic China. *Proc Nat Acad Sci* **101**(51), 17593–17598, at 17593.

[50] Cheese-making dates back almost as far as beer-production. See McClure SB, Magill C, Podrug E, *et al.* (2018). Fatty acid specific δ13C values reveal earliest Mediterranean cheese production 7,200 years ago. *PLoS One*, **13**(9), e0202807. See also "Evidence of 7,200-year-old cheese-making found on the Dalmatian Coast," *Phys Org News*, September 5, 2018, https://phys.org/news/2018-09-earliest-mediterranean-cheese-production-revealed.html

[51] Bacteria in cheese break down some of the lactose as the cheese ages. "Aged" cheese, like Parmesan, Gouda, and "sharp" cheddar, are typical examples.

cheese, varies according to where it is made and the various means of processing it.[52] So, in effect, beer-making — like so many other food-related technologies — reflects humans' ability to adapt.

Archaeologists found 13,000-year-old beer residues in a cave, associated with Natufian mortuary rituals, near Haifa, Israel.[53] This is a *really* long time ago to be "brewing" beer, and one might reasonably ask, "How did these Neolithic humans do it?" Li Liu explains the basic process:

> Ancient brewing processes had great regional variations [citations omitted], but would have involved three basic stages. 1. Malting: grains are germinated in water, drained, dried, and then stored for use. 2. Mashing: the malt is coarsely ground or crushed in a container, mixed with water, and heated until the temperature reached to and maintained in the range of 65°C–70°C over a period of time around 30 min to 4 h. 3. Fermenting: yeast is added to, or naturally settled on the wort [the infusion of ground malt or other grain before fermentation], the brewing container is covered with a lid, and the wort is allowed to sit for one or more days until the fermentation is completed.[54]

Of course, the Natufians would have needed grinding equipment and fermentation utensils. But as the research demonstrates,

---

[52] The website for "Two Frays Brewery in Pittsburgh" examines the different "styles" of beer and ale, based on their specific ingredients and how they are made. See https://www.twofraysbrewery.com/what-makes-one-beer-different-from-another

[53] See Liu L, Wang J, Rosenberg D, *et al*. Fermented beverage and food storage in 13,000 y-old stone mortars at Raqefet Cave, Israel: Investigating Natufian ritual feasting, supra; *Times of Israel*, September 12, 2018, 13,000-year-old brewery discovered in Israel, the oldest in the world, https://www.timesofisrael.com/13000-year-old-brewery-discovered-in-israel-the-oldest-in-the-world/

[54] Liu, supra, at 785.

they had them. The time and effort required to manufacture these items "indicate[s] an important ritual function played by alcoholic beverages in the Natufian culture."[55] Natufians found means to transform starch into beer.[56] They established parameters for this process, which have lasted for millennia.[57]

It is worth noting Liu's observation that "yeast is added to or naturally settled on the wort." Not every yeast is effective in transforming the carbohydrate in grain into ethanol. If such yeasts were not on the grains' surface, they would have had to come from another source, such as fruits with wild yeasts on their skins. Discovering this source would, itself, have been remarkable for a people with no idea of chemistry (it was not until 1857 that Louis Pasteur discovered that the yeast present on grape skins was responsible for fermentation).

A study provocatively called "Uncorking the past: Alcoholic fermentation as humankind's first biotechnology," discusses a drink dating to Early Neolithic China (~7000–6000 B.C.E.), which combined mead (a fermented beverage made from honey), rice beer, and a fruit wine made from grapes or hawthorn fruit (called "haws"). Jars containing the drink were placed so that the dead could imbibe.[58] Yet why did these early brewers make such a complex drink, mixing honey, grain, and fruit? The answer, again, probably lies in a type of primitive "biotech." Commenting on the challenges faced by brewers with no knowledge of chemistry, Muessdoerffer

---

[55] Liu, 792.

[56] See Liu's detailed explanation of the chemistry.

[57] Muessdoerffer, supra, identifies malting, mashing, and fermentation as the three basic steps of beer-making.

[58] McGovern P. (2020) Uncorking the past: Alcoholic fermentation as humankind's first biotechnology, in *Alcohol and Humans: A Long Social Affair*, Hockings K & Dunbar B (eds.). Oxford, 81–92.

observes: "As conversion of starch to sugar (malting) was poorly perfected initially, either additional fermentable sugars had to be added in the form of juices or honey and/or microorganisms capable of liquefying starch with exoenzymes had to be present to ensure fermentation."[59] In the Chinese mixture, honey and fruit would have served as a fermentable sugar source — with yeast on the fruit's skin — probably discovered through serendipity (we have no evidence of all the experiments that failed).[60] It is no wonder, then, that (even much later) "mixed beverages were widespread throughout Roman-Hellenistic times and the Middle Ages."[61]

The skills required for brewing were developed independently in widely disparate geographical areas. In the Fertile Crescent, the Sumerians (~ 2000 B.C.E.) worshipped a goddess of brewing, Ninkasi, who not coincidentally was also the goddess of harvesting (and of lovemaking and war, but that's another story). A long poem, the *Hymn to Ninkasi*, contains a recipe for beer-making that, not surprisingly, requires the addition of honey and wine before fermentation. A line in the poem states that beer "makes the liver happy and fills the heart with joy." The Sumerian

---

[59] Muessdoerffer, 4.

[60] McGovern, supra, states that while the evidence revealed no visible trace of (highly volatile) alcohol, "fermentation of the mixed ingredients, however, can be inferred, because the 'wine yeast' (*Saccharomyces cerevisiae*) occurs in honey and on the skins of sugar-rich fruits," 17597. On the repeated "experiments" of these Neolithic brewers, Stefan Estreicher states: "Even though the Neolithic people who lived at that site did not understand yeast or fermentation, they obviously figured out the necessary processes, and probably optimized them. The complex combination of ingredients also suggests that this was not their first fermented beverage." Estreicher S. (2017) The beginning of wine and viticulture. *Phys Status Solidi C* **14**(7), 1700008, 1.

[61] Muessdoerffer, 5.

Epic of Gilgamesh (~2100 B.C.E., with a more complete version ~1200 B.C.E.) features a wild man, Enkidu, who drinks seven jugs of beer and starts to sing joyfully.

When the Babylonians conquered the Sumerians, and imposed the *Code of Hammurabi*, it recorded twenty kinds of beer.[62] It also regulated the price and strength of beer.[63] In ancient Egypt, workers who built the pyramids were paid in beer.[64] The brewing process was displayed on the walls of tombs, where beer played a role in worship and medical practice.[65] But here's a question: what did the Egyptians do, surrounded by desert, with no grapes handy to provide necessary yeasts? In fact, there *were* grapes, which were grown on vines that climbed trellises or trees.[66] The Egyptians might also have turned to dates or other fruits. However, evidence from beer residues suggests that in most cases, "a special type of bread or sour dough was used as a source of yeast."[67] This practice was the obverse of adding beer-yeast to make bread.

Today, the Real Food Encyclopedia states that "Beer is food."[68] But whatever you think of that claim, it would have received no pushback in 1000 B.C.E. As Rod Phillips explains:

---

[62] Andreas, supra, at 16, citing Smith G. (2014) *Beer: A Global History*. Reaktion Books, 7–11.

[63] Phillips R. (2014) *Alcohol: A History*. University of North Carolina Press, 18.

[64] Andreas, 17.

[65] Some beers were brewed specifically for religious purposes. One was intended for the gods who guarded Osiris' shrine, or their priests. See Lutz HF. (1922) *Viticulture and Brewing in the Ancient Orient*. JC Hinrich. Beer was also considered to be an effective laxative and purgative. See Phillips, 18.

[66] Wall paintings depict workers treading the grapes, holding onto straps so as not to fall into the juice.

[67] Muessdoerffer, 7.

[68] See Foodprint, https://foodprint.org/real-food/beer/

> [I]n the ancient world . . . [beer] was remarkably nutritious. The malting process raised the caloric value of the base cereal, giving beer more calories than bread made with an equivalent amount of grain. In addition, beer was rich in carbohydrates, vitamins, and proteins. It also gave its drinker a pleasant feeling. Although we cannot know for certain the alcohol level in ancient beer, it was probably high enough to make ab impact but not so high that drinking a liter or two a day — making it excellent for hydration — would prevent anyone from getting on efficiently and safely with daily life.[69]

Beer's nutritional value explains why, in effect, it was used as currency to pay pyramid builders. Yet in ancient Egypt, everyone drank beer, not just workers. Wall paintings of banquets depict consumption of what was likely beer *and* wine — beer from larger vessels, indicating larger quantities. Of course, regardless of class, alcoholic beverages were safer than water, which, for a variety of reasons, could be polluted.

But what was this ancient beer like? Not like anything we are familiar with. It was cloudy, i.e., unfiltered; often a mixture of barley and fruits or honey (though sometimes wheat, millet, or rye were used); and you drank it from "large jars through straws or tubes, probably to prevent the drinker from ingesting the husks and stalks that floated on the surface."[70] Drinkers were closer to the sources of their drink than when we open a pull-top can. If they were farmworkers, they may have harvested the ingredients.

The Greeks under Alexander the Great conquered Egypt in 331 B.C.E. and installed the Ptolemies (Macedonian-Greek

---

[69] Phillips, 18.

[70] Phillips, 18.

dynasty that ruled from 305 to 30 B.C.E.). They imposed a tax on beer and were suspicious of the fermentation process. Later, the Greeks denounced beer as making men effeminate; in accordance with Hippocrates' humoral theory of medicine that sorted substances into hot, cold, dry, and wet, wine was hot and thus male, while beer was cold and female.[71] Though the Romans picked up on the Greeks' preference, their legions marched through areas lacking a robust wine culture and had to be provisioned with beer. Roman shopping lists discovered in Britain include items for beer.

In the first century C.E., the Roman historian Tacitus commented that among the German tribes, "a liquid can be made from barley or wheat . . . having been corrupted [fermented]."[72] The old English epic poem, *Beowulf* (7th/8th century), set in 6th-century Scandinavia, has vivid scenes of ale and beer drinking that capture its importance in Anglo-Saxon society — reinforcing courage and promoting conviviality.[73] The characters, mostly of the nobility and warrior class, celebrate with feasting and by drinking beer and ale.[74] Contemporaneously, when the Vikings invaded Britain (late 8th century), they drank ale and mead, and were so fond of

---

[71] Phillips, 31; Muessdoerffer, 8.

[72] Tacitus, *On the Origin and Situation of the Germans*, **23**, 1.

[73] For example, when Unferth insults Beowulf, Beowulf responds: "Well, friend Unferth, you have had your say/abut Breca and me. But it was mostly beer/that was doing the talking." *Beowulf*, ll. 530–531. Trans. Heaney S. (2012) *Norton Anthology of English Literature*. Norton.

[74] There is a special drinking cup in *Beowulf*, passed around as an expression of unity. The scene is paradigmatic. As McGovern remarks in "Fermented beverages of pre- and proto-historic China," "Rulers and 'upper class' individuals with leisure and resources particularly were drawn to feasting on a grand scale, which often featured special fermented beverages served in and drunk from special vessels," id. at 17593.

drinking that, as Andreas remarks, they "even managed to brew beer on board their longships during raiding campaigns."[75]

Yet the Vikings were hardly unique. Ale-drinking was common among medieval warriors. On long marches, where water could become contaminated, alcoholic beverages replaced it. During the siege of Dover Castle in 1216, about 1000 soldiers consumed 20,000 gallons of ale over 40 days, along with copious amounts of wine.[76] Did such consumption affect the nature of warfare? Depending on the strength of the drink, it could have.

Evidence of the use of hops dates from the 8th, 9th, and 10th centuries. Monasteries in France and Germany were centers of brewing and had statutes addressing hops, sometimes as payment of tithes. Remains from a Viking place of trade on the German coast reveal the use of hops. Muessdoerffer states that "hop residues were detected in high numbers in the remains of a cargo vessel from the 9th century at Graveney on the English coast. Thus, it can be assumed that hops were in use outside the monasteries and even traded between the continent and the British Isles.[77] This commodification of hops — in Germany, in England — reflects its rising use: enough was traded that you could make money off it. Who would have bought it in these quantities? Professional brewers. Unlike monasteries, they sold beer commercially; their output competed with that of other brewers.

The resulting competition enforced communal standards set by professional guilds that were subject to government regulation. These guilds arose in northern Europe during the 13th century and were urban phenomena; large-scale production (i.e., at a scale that greatly exceeded even the largest household's) needed a

[75] Andreas, 19.

[76] Phillips, supra, 78.

[77] Moessdoerffer, 11.

concentrated customer base. By the 16th century, brewers' guilds were found in most European cities. Governments began taxing commercially produced beer and issued regulations affecting concerns such as additives and pricing. They regulated beer consumption to ensure sufficient grain supply for baking bread (especially during Europe's repeated famines).

Beer began to supplant ale because of its greater longevity. Ale, which was made without hops, would spoil after a few weeks; beer could last for months. As Hannah Glasse's cookbook suggests, ale was more of a home brew. In 1492, Henry VIII established a dedicated brewery to supply his ships with beer. Beer was at least as popular as ale among pub-goers. By the 16th century, the British military drank only beer.[78] In the 17th century, Samuel Pepys, the Secretary of the Admiralty, decreed that every sailor should receive a gallon of beer per day. By the 18th century, beer-drinking segued into a truculent nationalism. Along with consuming quantities of red meat (even for breakfast), it symbolized Britons' masculine prowess:

> The French with their vineyards are meager and pale
> They drink of the squeezings of half ripen'd fruit;
> But we, who have hop-grounds to mellow our ale,
> Are rosy and plump, and have freedom to boot . . .
>
> Should the French dare invade us, thus arm'd with our poles,
> We'll bang their bare ribs, make their lanthern-jaws ring;
> But your beef eating, beer drinking, Britons are souls
> Who will shed their last drop for their country and king.[79]

---

[78] Andreas, 21.

[79] From *The Scots Nightingale . . . A New and Select Collection of the Best Scots and English Songs* (1779), 164. The British attitude was starkly opposite to the Greeks' concern that beer-drinking was effeminate.

When George Cheyne's *An Essay on Health and Long Life* (1724) claimed that water was sufficient for human needs, he was widely condemned. Defenders of beer and ale claimed that these beverages were necessary not just for soldiers, but for workingmen. Everyone drank beer and ale, even for breakfast. This included women, as evidenced in Mary Collier's *The Woman's Labour* (1739)

> At length bright *Sol* illuminates the Skies
> And summons drowsy Mortals to arise;
> Then comes our Mistress to us without fail,
> And in her Hand, *perhaps*, a Mug of Ale
> To cheer our Hearts, and also to inform
> Herself, what Work is done that very Morn.

This Mistress probably brewed her own ale (or, more likely, her servants did). But given the importance of beer and ale — not just as a drink, but in the case of ale as a baking necessity — the challenge was how to manage the brewing process. It could be tricky.

Several DIY manuals emerged in the fiercely competitive market for self-help books. Samuel Child's *Everyman His Own Brewer* (1790) went through nine editions, after an earlier title by the same name (1768). There was George Watkins' *The Compleat Brewer; Or, the Art and Mystery of Brewing* (1760, 1767, 1773). William Ellis' *The London and Country Brewer* (1734) went through seven editions, and the earlier *Guide to Gentlemen and Farmers for Brewing Malt-Liquors* (1703) went through five. These and similar texts marketed themselves energetically.[80]

[80] For an extensive discussion of 18th-century brewing manuals, see Sherman S. (2010) *Invention of the Modern Cookbook*. Greenwood.

In effect, they promoted an alternative to tea-drinking, which was said to cause weakness. Tea and toast for breakfast, instead of ale and steak, was maligned as effeminate.

But home-brewing became increasingly quaint. By the 18th century, brewing was fast becoming industrialized. In effect, it was one more outcrop of the Industrial Revolution. In Britain, the first steam-powered brewery opened in 1784. London became the center of large-scale brewing, offering a vast population of drinkers. Vats became enormous. In 1790, one vat held 10,000 barrels.[81] Muessdoerffer observes that "When such a vat collapsed in 1814, 7600 barrels of porter [a thick, dark beer] flooded the brewery and its neighborhood, destroying several houses and killing eight people."[82] To service this level of production, there had to be commensurate storage facilities and transportation, as well as financing. An activity that was once local and home-based, was fast becoming integrated with the nation's infrastructure. While DIY manuals bullishly marketed themselves to home-brewers, the mega-brewers were drawing away their potential readers with massive marketing efforts of their own.

Of course, large-scale brewing spread throughout Europe. It became a science, for example, with the introduction of the thermometer and the development of reliable methods to measure and control the conversion of sugars into ethanol. Beer could be standardized, from one mammoth batch to the next. In a 1876 essay, *Etudes sur la Biere*, Louis Pasteur recommended that yeasts be purified of bacteria.

---

[81] Compare the mammoth "digesters" used in late 18th-century soup kitchens, capable of reducing an entire cow to soup. See Sherman S, supra, *Imagining Poverty*. The soup kitchen industrialized the process of feeding the poor.

[82] Muessdoerffer, 24.

After the Civil War, American industrialization boomed. Though, as in Europe, beer and ale production had started as a home-based local activity, that changed — albeit more slowly, due to the country's sparse population. Beers included native grains such as corn and rice and, in this sense, became distinctly American. In the Massachusetts Bay Colony, John Winthrop won a prize for his corn-based brew. Immigrants made enormous contributions because, in effect, virtually everyone was an immigrant. American beers reflected their respective heritages — starting with the Pilgrims, who advised later immigrants to bring malt with them to ensure their beer supplies. Soon after the country was settled, there were breweries. Manhattan got its first brewery in 1632 (while it was still Dutch); by 1637, there was one in Massachusetts Bay, and there was one in Rhode Island in 1638. William Penn built a brewhouse in 1683.

In 1789, to promote industry and discourage the consumption of hard liquor, Massachusetts passed a law encouraging the manufacture and consumption of beer. In part, it acted because American beer was still considered inferior. This changed over time, especially after the introduction of American lager — first produced by a German immigrant, John Wagner, in 1840. But think about it: where Europe and the rest of the world had thousands of years to perfect their beer-making techniques, the Americans made enormous strides in a few hundred. Really, not at all bad. Of course, they benefited from European experience, but they also developed distinctive American beers.

Wine

The previous section discussed a complex fermented beverage made of grain, honey, and fruit, where the fruit (along with the honey) contributed to fermentation. This beverage, almost certainly alcoholic, was the product of expedience; the grain would not have fermented on its own *but for the fruit* (unless wild yeasts had landed on it). Technically, the archaeologists who found this mixture identified the fruit-based component as "fruit wine," though they reported no evidence that this so-called wine had ever been a stand-alone product that would have been drunk on its own. So, in this section on wine, we will focus on fermented beverages made deliberately and exclusively from fruit and, more particularly, from grapes — and that would be consumed as such.[83] This type of wine still goes way back in history but would be identifiable as "wine" by anyone living today.

Archaeological evidence demonstrates that grape wine was produced as early as 6000–5800 B.C.E. in the South Caucasus, in an area that is now Georgia, bordering the Black Sea, Russia, Turkey, and Azerbaijan.[84] Previously, the earliest evidence for grape wine was from northwestern Iran, 5400–5000 B.C.E. But wine drinking was not isolated. There is evidence for a trade in wine, emanating from Iraq and Iran, from ~3500 B.C.E.

---

[83] In "The beginning of wine and viticulture," supra, at 1, Estreicher limits "wine" to "the result of the intentional fermentation of *Vitis vinifera* grapes [the common grape vine]." Patrick McGovern observes that *Vitis vinifera*, as domesticated from the wild Eurasian grape, "became the basis of widespread 'wine culture' throughout the Near East and Egypt," ultimately spreading to most of the world. See McGovern P, Jalabadze M, Batiuk S, *et al.* (2017). Early neolithic wine of Georgia in the South Caucasus. *Proc Nat Acad Sci* **114**(48), E10309–E10318, at 10309. On the complexities of cultivating wild grapes, see Renfrew JM. (2003) Archaeology and the origin of wine production, in *Wine: A Scientific Exploration*, Sandler M & Pinder R (eds.). Routledge, 57–69.

[84] McGovern P, Jalabadze M, Batiuk S, *et al.* (2017) Early neolithic wine of Georgia in the South Caucasus. *Proc Nat Acad Sci* **114**(48), E10309–E10318.

Ancient Egypt produced its own wine. T.G.H. James states that "The evidence for wine production from the very start of the historic period — the beginning in the 1st Dynasty in about 3000 B.C. — is incontrovertible, although its interpretation depends much on what is known of later practice.[85] This need to "interpret" the evidence arises from an insufficient development in the hieroglyphic script. Accordingly, his study includes an extensive examination of recovered wine jars, as well as of wine-making scenes from excavated tombs.

J.M. Renfrew cites pictorial evidence of wine production on tomb walls from the Old (mid- to late 3rd millennium B.C.E.) and Middle Kingdoms (slightly later) where "the processes depicted include picking the grapes, treading them, several men pressing the residues through a cloth by twisting it using poles to get more purchase, bottling it, and sealing the bottles."[86] King Tut's tomb contained 26 wine jars, all meticulously labeled as to the vineyard's location, its ownership, the year, and the name of the chief winemaker. So, was Tut an early wine snob?[87] He was probably at least eclectic in his tastes. As James points out, "wines of different qualities from different sources were drunk by the higher ranks of

---

[85] See James TGH. (2003) The earliest history of wine and Its importance in ancient Egypt, in *The Origins and Ancient History of Wine: Food and Nutrition in History and Anthropology*, McGovern PE, Fleming SJ, & Katz SH (eds.). Routledge, 197–214, at 198.

[86] Renfrew, supra, at 61.

[87] The labeling of wine jars was a common practice at least 200 years before Tut. See James TGH, supra. So, Tut may have been less snobbish than curious. As Leonard Lesko observes, "The inscriptions on the 26 wine jars . . . contain better information than many of the labels on today's best bottles." See Lesko, Egyptian wine production during the new kingdom, in McGovern, supra, *Origins*, 215–230, at 221.

society . . . and were thought to be suitable constituents among the necessities for a good afterlife."[88]

Of course, the general population was less concerned with specific vintages. They most likely drank ale. Still, they would have cared about wine's medicinal usefulness. The Ebers medical papyrus, ~1500 B.C.E., demonstrates that wine was used in restoring appetite and strength. There is also evidence that it was used in enemas, bandaging (the alcohol would have been an antiseptic), and to reduce swelling in limbs.[89]

Wine was also important to religious practice. At the end of the New Kingdom, Rameses III made huge offerings of wine to the gods. In a section of the Harris papyrus (late second century B.C.E.), he reminds the god Amun that he created vineyards for him in the north and south and equipped them with vintners and slaves. The association of wine and religion goes way back in cultural history. In the Judeo/Christian tradition, scholars have long pondered the influence of Egyptian life and religion on the Old Testament.[90]

The Old Testament reveals in broad outline how people lived — and made a living — during the time it was written. It's very interesting on the place of wine in Mesopotamian culture. Consider the story of Noah, which scholars date to ~1000–500 B.C.E., though some consider its origins in Mesopotamian flood mythology from perhaps 1000 years earlier. Genesis 9:20–21 states:

---

[88] James, supra, 204.

[89] Renfrew, 77.

[90] See, e.g., Ebeling JR, Wright JE, Elliott MA, *et al.* (eds.). (2017) *The Old Testament in Archaeology and History*. Baylor University Press, Waco, Texas; Hassan FA. (2010) Egypt in the memory of the world. *Egyptian Archaeol* **259**, 273.

20 And Noah began to be an husbandman, and he planted a vineyard;
21 And he drank of the wine, and was drunken . . .

A "husbandman" was a farmer, and, after the flood, Noah planted grapes. In the time between verses 20 and 21, the grapes were harvested and made into wine, which caused Noah to get drunk. In the Bible's chronology, Noah was the first vintner and the first person to drink so much that he got intoxicated. The chronology further reveals that 726 years elapsed between Adam's death and the flood[91]: the story's authors want us to understand that wine appeared many years after humanity's fall. Those years, characterized by continued sin, resulted in the flood and almost universal death. So, what is the role of wine in these events? Some rabbis argue that it is to signify God's mercy, in that by introducing wine-making after the flood, Noah offers humanity relief from the burden of work it inherited because of Adam's fall. Of course, what matters from our perspective is that wine production was recognized in ancient Mesopotamia (modern-day Iraq, Syria, and Turkey) as much as 2500 to 3500 years ago.

While we associate wine with the New Testament (100–200 C.E.), where Jesus turns water into wine (John 2:1–11), the Old Testament — more than 1000 years older — contains multiple references to wine. For example, David carries a bottle of wine so "that such as be faint in the wilderness may drink" (2 Samuel 16:1–2). Psalm 104:15 cites "wine that maketh glad the heart of man;" in Judges 9:13, wine "cheereth God and man" (wine-drinking is one way that man is *like* God); Proverbs 31:6 commands: "Give . . . wine unto those that be of heavy hearts," suggesting that

---

[91] The span of 726 years is based on biblical chronology provided in Genesis.

wine offers comfort. The Old Testament also inflects wine with prophetic significance. Amos 9:13 predicts that in days to come "the mountains shall drop sweet wine," while Isaiah 25:6 predicts that God shall "make unto all people . . . a feast of wines on the lees." Wine doesn't just enhance happiness; it helps define future happiness. It is a marker of hope.

But when drinking leads to drunkenness, wine is a vehicle for regression — literally, for re-enacting the fall. After Noah gets drunk, his son finds him "uncovered within his tent" (Genesis 9:21–22), in a version of Adam's nakedness after eating the apple (Genesis 3:7). It's hard to miss the allusion — the parallel, albeit on a smaller scale. But Noah is not unique in over-indulging. Proverbs 20:1 declares: "Wine is a mocker, strong drink is raging: and whosoever is deceived thereby is not wise." Proverbs 23:20 admonishes: "Be not among winebibbers; among riotous eaters of flesh." Proverbs 31:4 cautions: ". . . It is not for kings to drink wine; nor for princes strong drink." Isaiah 5:11-12 insists that excessive wine-drinking amounts to dissipation and is tantamount to sin:

> 5:11 Woe unto them that rise up early in the morning, that they may follow strong drink; that continue until night, till wine inflame them.
>
> 5:12: After the harp, and the viol, the tabret, and pipe, and wine are in their feasts; but they regard not the work of the LORD, neither consider the operation of his hands.

The verses from Isaiah hint at a type of depressive, solo drinking, followed by debauchery.

Wine could also be an instrument of trickery. In Genesis 19:30–38, Lot's daughters muddle his senses with wine so that he impregnates them without recognizing that he is committing incest.

All these references (and others, e.g., to wine presses) amplify the fact that when the Old Testament was written (~1400 B.C.E. to 400 B.C.E.), wine was produced and consumed in the Near East. People got drunk. The poor probably had less access to wine and so would have been limited to ale or some mixed alcoholic beverage (though the Old Testament does not explicitly cite such a limitation). Still, it prescribes a schema for *how* to consume wine (and alcohol in general) that is meant to be applicable universally.

Of course, the Mesopotamians were not the only people in this period familiar with wine. As we noted in our discussion of beer, the ancient Greeks privileged wine, regarding it as "hot" under Herodotus' theory of humors. Thus, it was a drink for males. It was the warriors' drink. In Book 9 of the *Odyssey* (8th century B.C.E.), Odysseus' men steal a store of wine from the Ciccones, who were Thracians allied with the Trojans. They also take the Ciccones' women as slaves. Both incidents are insults and reflect the hyper-masculinized violence of the Trojan War. As Iain Gately observes, in ancient Greece, "wine was the drink of fighting men, the indispensable lubricant of their culture of death and honor, of sacking cities, of carrying off armor, cattle, and women. All their rituals were punctuated with libations of wine — otherwise, the gods did not pay attention."[92]

Yet there was another side to the Greeks' wine drinking. As Thibaut Boulay demonstrates, the Greeks had developed an elaborate wine aesthetic.[93] Such "wine-tasting," however, was not an early version of our current wine-snobbery. Rather, it reflected the

---

[92] Gately I. (2008) *Drink: A Cultural History of Alcohol*. Penguin, 12.

[93] Boulay T. (2015) Wine appreciation in ancient Greece, *A Companion to Food in the Ancient World*, 273–282.

idea that wine (as a hot beverage) was medicinal; it was nourishing, and choosing the right wine, based on various aesthetic factors, was like designing an effective medical/nutritional regimen. For example, "the color, taste, consistency, bouquet, and age of wines allowed distinctions to be made in choosing a remedy for some physical ailments, or to retain or restore the balance of humors."[94] Wines could be classified by their qualities, adapted to various diseases and conditions. If, as was assumed, the old were cold and dry, the right wine might be restorative.

Based on such consideration, an "eonological discourse developed" involving "a refined, elaborate, and codified art of wine tasting."[95] Wines were examined based on several complementary factors, for example, their look (usually based on color), bouquet, consistency, and taste. So, for example, commenting on the various colors of wine, Athenaeus observes that:

> Among the wines, there are white wine, claret wine, and dark wine. White is by its nature the lightest, diuretic, and hot, and, because it promotes digestion; it sets the head on fire; indeed, this wine tends to rise upwards. Dark wine, when it is not sweet, is the most nourishing and astringent, but even when it is sweet, it is more nutritious than white or claret wine.[96]

The passage, citing the medicinal and nutritional aspects of wine, sounds like some modern "wellness" dictum. It turns the reputed hotness of wine — its ability to fire up maleness and truculent behavior — toward helping the drinker with everyday (and

---

[94] Boulay, 274.

[95] Boulay, 274.

[96] Athenaeus. Fl. 2nd–3rd century, C.E. Cited, in Boulay, 274–275.

non-gendered) physical concerns, i.e., digestion and improving one's diet. Lighter wines, with less alcohol and residual sugar, were recommended for heart disease.

This approach to wine-tasting — as primarily an adjunct to medicine — is striking. Though wine had long been regarded as nourishing and as a remedy for an array of ailments,[97] the Greeks refined this straightforward approach. For them, the effectiveness of wines was hinged to aesthetic judgments based on color, taste, bouquet, consistency, and the resulting degree of heat. It wasn't enough just to say, "Wine can [some ameliorating verb]." Instead, one had to stop, analyze a particular wine in several sensory dimensions, and then say, "This wine, with these characteristics [some ameliorating verb]."

Boulay examines the complex olfactory and taste-related dimensions of wine. These were broken down into an array of sub-categories. Regarding taste, there was sweet, unctuous, sharp, astringent, harsh, acid, salty, and bitter (not unfamiliar to modern gastronomes). These categorizations, as developed in contemporary treatises, "allow categorization of wines according to their therapeutic virtues, in a terminology outside the field of hedonistic taste."[98] They represent one of those instances where something from the past feels familiar — when Noah gets drunk, we get the picture — but really is not. So, while we might recommend an astringent wine to accompany a fatty, marbled steak or a chocolate dessert, it was, to the Greeks, thought to soothe the

---

[97] See, for example, the Ebers papyrus, supra. See generally, Norrie PA. (n.d.) The history of wine as a medicine, in *Wine: A Scientific Exploration*, supra, 21–55.

[98] Boulay, 279.

stomach. Likewise, Galen held that sweet wine flavored with thyme (a hot and dry plant) was "indicated for poor digestion, torpor of the nerves, winter chills, and venomous animals."[99]

Of course, while all these categories gave Greek wine drinkers what Boulay calls an "interpretive framework," it hardly restricted their imaginations or appreciation of wine. Wine-tasting was still subjective, even if an expert presumed to define a wine's dominant qualities. So, what seemed bitter to one person might seem pleasantly astringent to another. Moreover, despite the coupling of wine's medical and aesthetic attributes, Greeks still got drunk.[100] What finally mattered was that the Greeks established a complex, multi-modal vocabulary for analyzing and describing wine, albeit the ultimate motivation was not mere enjoyment. This vocabulary, reflecting a respect for wine, represented a cognitive advance over other cultures' relationship to wine-drinking.

By the time of Hippocrates (5th–4th centuries B.C.E.) and Galen (1st–2nd centuries C.E.), the Greeks had long been familiar with wine. J. M. Renfrew observes that domesticated grapevines were found in northern Greece dating from ~2500 B.C.E.; on Crete, wine-making from wild grapes was found to date from ~3000 B.C.E.[101] Remains on mainland Greece from ~1600 to 1200 B.C.E,. consisting of large storage vessels, indicate the "great importance of wine," which, along with olive oil, was exported to "Syria, Palestine, Egypt, Cyprus, and even as far west as Sicily and

---

[99] Id.

[100] Drinking in Ancient Greece, https://warwick.ac.uk/news/knowledgecentre/arts/classics-ancient-history/drinking-greece

[101] Renfrew JM. (2002). Archaeology and the origins of wine production, in *Wine*. CRC Press, 56–69, 62.

southern Italy."[102] During this period, wine was used in initiation ceremonies, as a status-marker, and even perhaps during business transactions (all of this seems uncannily familiar).[103]

What's interesting is that in later, classical times — that is, around the time of Hippocrates — Greeks became ambassadors of wine: they not only cultivated vines, "but also spread the practice of viticulture to Sicily, southern Italy (which they called 'Oenotria,' the land of trained vines), the southern France and to their colonies on the Black Sea as far as the Crimea." Areas that today boast of "terroir," must still trace the *practice* of viticulture back to Greece. Of course, even 2500 years ago, wines varied. Greek colonies, e.g., Massilia (the ancient name for Marseille), made their own distinctive wines.

Greek wines were often flavored with aromatic herbs (a kind of Greek vermouth!) or blended with other wines (not unlike modern Bordeaux). Renfrew observes that "wine was almost always drunk diluted with water,"[104] though — apart from making it harder to get drunk — this may have been a way for alcohol to disinfect water (which, at least in urban areas, could easily have been polluted).

The Romans imported Greek wine, which dominated the market, though by the early first millennium, Rome began mass-producing wine itself to serve the demand of urban areas. Large wineries were "owned by financiers, managed by stewards, and

---

[102] Renfrew, 63.

[103] For an excellent summary of wine's refinement and expansion across a swath of areas adjacent to the Mediterranean, see Harutyunyan M & Malfeito-Ferreira M. (2022) The rise of wine among ancient civilizations across the Mediterranean basin. *Heritage* **5**(2), 788–812.

[104] Renfrew, 64

run by slaves."[105] There were bars in Pompeii, Herculaneum, and Ostia. Wine was a business. Wine merchants owned specially designed ships which plied the Tiber, carrying wine in amphorae; by the second and third centuries, barrels and casks replaced them. While huge amounts of Spanish wine were imported, large amounts of wine were shipped to areas in Gaul (now France); later in the millennium, these areas developed their own vineyards. Eventually, wine production shifted east.

Amidst all this activity, the Romans developed an early system designating the relative quality of wines produced in different regions. These categories (based essentially on taste) differed from those of the Greeks, for whom taste was primarily *instrumental*, and quality was measured primarily by the effect of a wine on one's health. Nonetheless, the Romans believed that wine had medicinal properties. It was a cure for depression, a laxative, a cure for halitosis and gout, and even a remedy for tapeworm. It was an everyday necessity; depending on a wine's quality, wine (of some sort) was available to everyone.

The Romans recognized drunkenness. In Seneca's *Moral Letters* (~65 C.E.), letter 83 inveighs against getting drunk, suggesting that it represents a wish to go mad. In his speeches, Cicero (1st century B.C.E.) called out drunkards as dangerous. So, while Noah's drunkenness is hidden from most people, Roman writers attack the spectacle of drunkenness — it is a public danger and disgrace.

There has been significant research into wine production and consumption during the Byzantine period, also known as that of the Eastern Roman Empire, which dates from the 4th century

105 Renfrew, 66.

B.C.E. (the dedication of Constantinople) to Constantinople's fall to the Ottomans in 1453.[106] The period is vast, as was the geography around the Mediterranean that it encompassed. It included the Crusades (1095–1291). Since the original Byzantines were Greek, wine was already a staple. In "Wine: Byzantium's Gift to the West," Ilias Anagnostakis states:

> In medieval times, both Constantinople and the empire itself were viewed as a place where wine flowed freely. Northern Europeans gave Constantinople the nickname Winbourg, the City of Wine.[107]

Between the 5th and 7th centuries, wine was traded between Byzantium and such distant places as the Caucasus, Crimea, Ireland, and England. In the 10th–12th centuries, Byzantine missionaries brought wine to newly Christianized areas, e.g., in Bulgaria, Serbia, and Russia, for their use in the Eucharist. Anagnostakis argues that "the contribution of monasteries and the church in general was a catalyst, therefore, not only for the dissemination and 'Christianization' of wine culture, but also for the evolution of the beverage and the symposia (drinking parties) of the ancient world into more morally acceptable forms of wine consumption." The pattern is consistent with the wine/religion nexus that had existed… more or less forever.

But there was blowback. The literary figure of the *krasopateras*, literally "wine father," or drunk monk, became a notorious (in)version of the supposedly ascetic monk. The figure became

---

[106] See, for example, Afaneh S. (2013) Embodiment of grape growing and wine manufacturing in the arts of the Roman and Byzantine Empires. *Ann Fac Arts Ain Shams Univ* **41**(January–March), 339–383.

[107] Anagnostakis I. (2016) Wine: Byzantium's gift to the West, https://www.greece-is.com/wine-byzantiums-gift-west/

so embedded in wine culture that, even today, it's easy to buy Krasopateras Red Wine.[108] There is a Krasopateras Grill House in Lamia, Greece, which, presumably, sells Greek wines. During the Byzantine period, the Empire's wines were known across Europe, particularly the sweet wine of Bithynia.[109] The area was the main supplier of wine to Constantinople, whose population preferred it to the watery, resin-infused product of vineyards from other areas.

In medieval Europe, wine was a crucial element of the Catholic Mass, and monasteries in France and Germany became large producers. The monks, such as the Benedictines and Cistercians, also brewed beer! Neither effort, however, was primarily for profit — the communities were supplying the Church, and (in the case of beer) looking after their own sustenance; beer was nutritious, and both were safer than water. Of course, members of the Church enjoyed drinking — perhaps to excess. In Geoffrey Chaucer's *Canterbury Tales* (late 14th century), the "Summoner's Tale" depicts a corrupt church official who reeks of garlic, leeks, onions, and whose pores exude strong red wine.

There was also plenty of wine outside the Church. The *Canterbury Tales* suggests that drunkenness was common; the "Pardoner's Tale" and "Miller's Tale" feature drunken characters.[110] The suggestion is that readers would have recognized them, although Chaucer is sufficiently detached to avoid any bludgeoning moralizing (which is why the *Tales* have lasted for 600 years).

---

[108] https://araxxon.com/products/krasopateras-rotwein-trocken-1-5l/

[109] Anagnostakis I. (2017) The sweet wine of Bithynia in the Byzantine era, in *Of Vines and Wines. The Production and Consumption of Wine in Anatolian Civilizations through the Ages*, Thys-Şenocak L. (ed.). Leuven, Peeters, 93–117.

[110] See *Moral Ambiguity in The Canterbury Tales*, https://digitalcommons.usu.edu/cgi/viewcontent.cgi?article=1751&context=honors

In the 16th century, Spanish missionaries took viticulture to Mexico and South America. By the 18th century, Spanish Franciscan missionaries had planted vineyards in California. So perhaps, in these monks' and missionaries' activities, there is the faint refraction of wine's role in so many earlier religious expressions. In any case, California now produces over 600 million gallons of wine a year, over 80% of the U.S.'s total production.

In 1630, the year that it was settled, the Massachusetts Bay Colony produced wine from native grapes. It petitioned the Massachusetts Bay Company, back in London, to send Frenchmen experienced in "planting of vines," though these experts never arrived.[111] In 1632, Governor John Winthrop secured a grant to plant a vineyard on Conant's Island in Boston Harbor. The wine, however, never materialized and was ultimately replaced by apples.

Distilled spirits

Any search for the origin of fermented beverages must rely on archaeological evidence dating back millennia. Neolithic Chinese, Mesopotamians, and ancient Greeks are in the mix. But it is different with distilled spirits, whose origin is relatively recent. Historians take over from archaeologists; they study printed texts (not old pots and wall paintings) along with relatively well-preserved production equipment. Their sources are in libraries (not caves or ruins); as to the equipment, it is cataloged at the Smithsonian. There's no need for radiocarbon dating. The whole subject feels modern (or proto-modern, anyway), at least when compared to the origins

[111] Pinney T. (1989) *A History of Wine in America, Volume 1: From the Beginnings to Prohibition*,Vol. 1. University of California Press.

of beer- and wine-making. There are no claims for the religious significance of gin. Any suggestions of medical utility, say for the "heat" imparted by whiskey or brandy, are quickly tempered by warnings against over-consumption.

Compare, for example, the Greeks' elaborate medicalization of wine with a blunt ordinance issued by the Holy Roman Empire in 1530, inveighing against drinking to one's health with distilled spirits: "The abuse and mischiefs of pledging healths has increased everywhere, becoming more and more entrenched and extensive, leading to blasphemy, murder, manslaughter, adultery, and other such misdeeds."[112] While we would object to lumping adultery with murder, the language still resonates with that mandated by the Alcoholic Beverage Act of 1988: "GOVERNMENT WARNING: . . . Consumption of Alcoholic Beverages impairs your ability to drive a car or operate machinery, and may cause health problems." By the early 16th century, "pledging healths" with alcohol was already understood as unhealthy, that is, by making one antisocial. By 1572, doctors in Germany were warning that "brandy is more seriously damaging than other [drinks, which were undistilled], especially to pregnant women and young working people, and causes many damaging illnesses and maladies on a daily basis."[113] This language anticipates another portion of the Alcoholic Beverage Act's required warning: "According to the Surgeon General, women should not drink alcoholic beverages during pregnancy because of the risk of birth defects." The statement from 1572 turns any medicalization of alcohol on its head — these physicians made judgments that we find relatable.

---

[112] Cited in Phillips, 116.

[113] Id., 116.

As Rod Phillips describes the timeline:

> Alcoholic beverages made by distillation appeared in Europe by the twelfth century, but even as late as 1500 they were produced in very limited quantities and almost exclusively for medical purposes. Yet by the end of the 1500s, distilled spirits had entered the mainstream of European and American drinking cultures and the bloodstreams of their populations. … It has been suggested that the first batch of spirits was produced in 1100, at the prestigious medical school at Salerno, in southern Italy, but if that is so, it took a remarkably long time for alcohol distilling to catch on more widely.[114]

The 16th century is no longer Geoffrey Chaucer's world, where most drunks were tipsy clerics. It broaches our own world.[115] So, after glancing at some Medieval work in medicinal distillation, we start our discussion in the Early Modern period (generally said to date from 1500 to 1800, and to include the Renaissance, Reformation, Age of Exploration, and Enlightenment, all of which some may claim were fueled by distilled spirits).

Distilled spirits developed relatively late because the associated technology is more complex. Think about it. Beer-making requires a pot and a yeast source; wine requires a rudimentary

---

[114] Phillips, *Alcohol: A History*, supra, 110–111. On the earliest history of distilled spirits, see DeSalle R, Tattersall I & Acevedo MA. (2022) *Distilled: A Natural History of Spirits*. Yale University Press; Phillips and Cockx L, Meloni G & Swinnen J. (2021) The water of life and death: A brief economic history of spirits. *J Wine Econ* **16**(4), 355–399.

[115] On concepts of habitual drunkenness and its treatment during this period, see Korostyshevsky D. (2022). Corrupting the body and mind: Distilled spirits, drunkenness and disease in early modern England and the British Atlantic world, in *Alcohol, Psychiatry and Society: Comparative and Transnational Perspectives, c. 1700–1990s*, 36–65.

press (or just foot-stomping) to extract the grape juice, and some barrels for aging; but distillation requires heating a fermented liquid to evaporate the alcohol, collecting the vapor, and then condensing the vapor (by means of specific cooling technology) back to a liquid with a higher concentration of alcohol. It might be repeated two or three times to further increase the concentration. You needed a still, as well as sufficient knowledge to use it. Both were hard to come by.

During the 12th and 13th centuries, European physicians and alchemists began experimenting with distilling alcohol for an elixir to treat stomach, kidney, and liver conditions, and, in general, the problems of aging. An early type of gin was developed in the 14th century and used as medicine against the Black Death that raged across Europe. Leonardo da Vinci designed an improved method for distilling alcohol, but only for use "as a solvent or an incendiary for military purposes"; he warned against drinking it.[116] However, these were rarefied efforts, largely restricted to the cognoscenti.

It took Johannes Gutenberg's invention of printing, around 1440, to make techniques for distilling alcohol accessible (at least to anyone who read Latin, which was most physicians).[117] Books on alchemy (a practice that relied on distillation) could be repurposed. The first printed book on distillation in the vernacular was by an Austrian physician: *A Very Useful Little Book on Distillations* (1476). In German, the *Little Book* provided recipes as well as insights into the technology. It was "a rampant best-seller," with 38 printings by 1500. It began to demystify distilling, and was the

---

[116] Phillips, 112.

[117] See Cockx, supra, on Latin texts from the 12th and 13th centuries that would, necessarily, have had limited circulation.

opening salvo in an accelerating process by which distilled alcohol would be transformed from medicine into a popular beverage. The Nuremberg authorities became so concerned that they banned home distilling.[118]

In 1500, a German physician published *Liber de Arte Distillandi: De Simplicibus* in Latin, claiming that alcohol cured an array of complaints from baldness to deafness and bad digestion. Before the 16th century, stills had been expensive, with access largely confined to physicians and monks (monasteries were still repositories of learning and would only start losing their position during the Reformation, which began in Germany in 1517 and spread to England in 1534). *Liber* implicitly recognizes that its audience was narrow, but it also helped promote the idea that (at least theoretically) its audience could expand. Sure enough, *Liber* was translated into English in 1527 as *The Virtuous Book of Distilling*, becoming one of the first works on science to be translated. The new title artfully shifts the emphasis on simplicity — which any manual might be expected to tout — to virtue. Distilling is good for you![119]

But by not literally translating the title, the English version obscures the original's objective. That is, by having designated distillation an "art," the *Liber* taps into Renaissance ideas that art encompasses a range of skilled, creative occupations beyond simple craftsmanship; an "art" is a more intellectual, refined practice.[120] Viewed in this light, the products of distillation — with

[118] De Salle & Tattersall, supra, at 37.

[119] The English translator states in his Preface that "Behold how much it exceeds to use medicine of efficacy natural by God ordained than wicked words or charms of efficacy unnatural by the devil invented."

[120] Well into the 17th century, the term "art" could be used to elevate the status of one who practiced an ostensibly humble profession. See, for example, Robert May's *The Accomplisht Cook: Or the Art and Mystery of Cookery* (1685).

increased alcoholic content — would exemplify the distiller's skill, which would enhance those products' value. Wouldn't some readers want to learn how to make them? Isn't pride perhaps even more of a motive than what's good for you?

Yet while *Liber* was the first printed book on an arc that traces distilled alcohol from medication to beverage, it was John French's *The Art of Distillation* (1651) that first clearly describes how to distill alcohol-containing liquids, e.g., from wine and fruits. His method of making "A Water Out of Berries" sets out the crucial, basic steps: first, steep the berries with sugar for three or four weeks, i.e., until they are fermented, then distill the mixture. He explains how to make "Spirit of Wine" from successive distillations that increase the spirit's strength. If you have never tried distillation, he provides detailed instructions and diagrams, as well as an extensive glossary of terms ("An Explanation of Such Hard Words and Terms of Art Which are Used in the Ensuing Treatise"). If you have never built a still, he shows you how, with specific instructions on the various types of vessels and furnaces. So, while *The Art* is laden with alchemical references (acknowledging the origin of distillation), and extols various "elixirs," it is an extremely practical manual, demonstrating how to build a still ("if [the furnace] be of forged iron or copper they must be coated inside, especially if you intend to use them for a strong fire") and use it to produce an array of beverages.

In a break from the Latin of alchemy, French wrote in the vernacular. Anyone could read him. He helped to pique public interest.[121] The market responded. By the early 18th century, books

---

[121] French's title, possibly a not-so-subtle reference to *Liber de Arte*, reinforces the idea that distilling is an art and success in it is a status marker. Accordingly, he cautions readers not to be presumptuous: "[I]f any artist would enter upon

in English eagerly advised readers on distilling spirits at home.[122] They assumed that households owned a still and that someone (probably the mistress or a servant) knew how to use it (or could learn).[123] For example, Thomas Tryon's expansively named *The way to get wealth: or a new and easie way to make twenty three sorts of wine . . . Also to make Cyder, Mead, Rum, Brandy, and Cordial waters* (1701), instructed readers on how to use honey, molasses, and sugar as a base, and even on how to distill spirits from the lees of wine. Hannah Wooley's *The Compleat Servant Maid* (1704) taught servants how to make Spirit of Roses, a rose-flavored liquor or cordial. The recipe is homely; no one needs to be a learned monk or physician to follow it; still, it encompasses every step from fermentation to distillation, and assumes that readers will understand these steps:

> Bruise the Rose in his own juice, adding thereto, being temperately warmed, in a convenient proportion, either of Yeast or Ferment; leave them a few days to ferment, till they get a strong and heady smell near like to Vinegar; then distill them, and draw so long as you find any scent of the Rose to come; then distill again so often

---

the practice of chemistry, let him apply himself to some expert artist for to be instructed in the manual operation of things, for by this means he will learn more in two months than he can by his practice and study in 7 years, as also avoid much pains and cost and redeem much time and cost which else of necessity he will lose."

[122] The genre is still going strong. See, e.g., O'Connor S. (2021) *The ABC's of Distilling: the Ultimate Guide to Making Your Own Vodka, Whiskey, Rum, Brandy, Moonshine, and More*. Andromeda Press; Malle B & Schmickl H. (2015) *The Artisan's Guide to Crafting Distilled Spirits*. Spikehorn Press.

[123] In the 18th century, the "still room" was a woman's domain. She was expected to teach relevant skills to the servants.

till you have purchased a perfect Spirit of Rose. You may also ferment the juice of Rose only, and after distill the same. (pp. 41–42).

By the 18th century, literacy among servants was growing. The frontispieces of cookbooks show them following the book as they cook. Books aimed at servants imparted skills, which (so it was claimed) would help them elevate their station. Distillation was obviously considered such a skill.

Still, distillation was hardly confined to the domestic sphere or, though they were declining, to monasteries. Lara Cockx observes that as early as the mid-17th century, "the growing demand for alcoholic distillation for drinking purposes stimulated private investments in distillation by wealthy individuals and alcohol production outside monasteries."[124] Perhaps the most recognizable feature of distillation's proto-modernity was its capture by proto-capitalism.

It is easy to understand investors' interest, even apart from the rising demand. Distillation increased the alcoholic content of wine and beer — if someone drank for the buzz, the buzz would come on faster. The higher alcohol content also inhibited spoilage (even adding hops to beer did not prevent its "turning" after a while). Distilled spirits could be transported longer distances.

Yet the rise of *individual* distilled spirits was uneven across Europe and the rest of the world. This was because of still another difference between wine-and-beer and the products of distillation, in that *types* of distilled spirits varied immensely depending on where they were made. Regional variations became even more pronounced based on variations in production technique.

For example, while areas that couldn't grow grapes *might* distill wine into brandy (as in Thomas Tryon's *The way to get wealth*),

[124] "The water of life and death," supra, at 7.

they might more easily make gin, a neutral grain spirit typically distilled from grain or barley and flavored with juniper. Likewise, rum was initially made in the Caribbean from abundant molasses, a byproduct of sugar refining; sugar was expensive in Europe, and remained so until demand increased in the 18th century with the rise of coffee-, tea-, and chocolate-drinking (the British did, however, play a role in blending and aging rum).[125] The French, of course, made cognac from the abundance of grapes and local wine. Whiskey was made from grain, and the types of whiskey varied according to the grain type (e.g., barley, corn, rye, wheat), fermentation and distilling techniques, aging process, and barrel type — each of these could be a treatise on their own.[126] Theoretically, whiskey could be made anywhere but, since the French were busy enough making cognac from wine, the Scots and Irish specialized in whiskey and malt whiskey. Vodka was made from cereal grains, but also from potatoes or sugar beets; though it could be made anywhere as well, Russia, Poland, Belarus, and Ukraine became the main producers.

America could make everything, and eventually it did. The only major spirit not produced (somewhere) in America is tequila, which is made from agave grown in Mexico (which regulates its production and branding). Yet because America *can* produce so much

---

[125] With the addition of sugar, tea, coffee, and chocolate were (for a while) rivals of distilled beverages, to which people also sometimes added sugar. The rivalry ceased, however, especially in Britain, once gin became a dominant drink.

[126] See, for example, Work HH. (2024) *Wood, Whiskey and Wine: A History of Barrels*. Reaktion Books; Gollihue J, Pook VG & DeBolt S. (2021) Sources of variation in bourbon whiskey barrels: A review. *J Inst Brew* **127**(3), 210–223; Reazin GH. (1981) Chemical mechanisms of whiskey maturation. *Am J Enol Vitic* **32**(4), 283–289.

"booze," production of any one type — e.g., bourbon or rum — varies according to changing tastes in domestic and export markets. For example, rum fell out of favor in recent years, but is now making a comeback, especially in the premium and craft sectors.

Back in the 17th and 18th centuries, however, as large-scale distillation replaced household and monastic production, it became enmeshed in macro-economics. For example, the Dutch imported brandy instead of making gin from home-grown grain because any such distillation risked creating a shortage of grain to make bread.[127] During the 17th century, known as the Dutch "Golden Age," the Dutch became among the earliest international spirits merchants — they not only imported brandy for their own use, but established stills in France for easier export.[128] So, while it is important to resist facile analogies, their practice of "off-shoring" is nonetheless recognizable in terms of globalization and, in that sense, it reflects still further on the "modernity" of distilled spirits.[129]

Great Britain was also globalizing.[130] In the 17th century, among its many imports were wine and cognac from France. But when it went to war with France in the late 17th century, most of

---

[127] See Cockx at 8. In our section on beer, above, we discuss a similar phenomenon in Great Britain when, during periods of scarcity, beer-making competed for the grain required by bakers.

[128] Id.

[129] As a 17th-century colonial power, the Dutch had an instinct for globalization, importing, and trading, in an array of products from colonies in Asia, Africa, and the Americas.

[130] Alexander Pope's *The Rape of the Lock* (1712–14) encapsulates Britain's trading prowess in lines describing imports adorning the dressing table of the poem's heroine: "Unnumber'd treasures ope at once, and here/The various off'rings of the world appear/ . . . This casket India's glowing gems unlocks/And all Arabia breathes from yonder box." See Canto I.

such imports ceased, and those that trickled in became subject to high tariffs. Consumption switched to Scotch and Irish whiskey, as well as Dutch gin. Beer production around London increased dramatically. Yet perhaps the most important development, with the most far-reaching consequences for how alcohol was perceived and understood, was that Parliament encouraged Britons to distill their own gin (which provided tax revenue at 2 pence/gallon).[131] By 1736, London had ~1500 stills.[132] The astonishing figure (about 1 per every 400 inhabitants) exemplifies what was known as the Gin Craze which, between 1700 and 1750, ostensibly held every man, woman, and child in Great Britain in thrall to gin. While it is unlikely that the entire population was under the influence, there was obvious panic (among those sober enough to care) that gin was causing widespread egregious behavior.[133]

Phillips, supra, explains the anxiety:

> [It] rested on the belief that gin was being abused not only by men, the traditional consumers to excess, but also — and especially — by women and children. Gin was called "Mother Gin" and "Mother Geneva," names that linked it to women and children. Mothers who guzzled gin were said to feed it to their older children to stop them complaining about being hungry, and indirectly to to their infants as they breast-fed.[134]

---

[131] There was a glut of grain in Britain at the time of Parliament's action. Encouraging the production of gin, made from grain, was a help to the land-owners. Additionally, distilling used up grain that was of insufficient quality for bread-baking. See Gately, 161.

[132] Phillips, supra, 124.

[133] For a nuanced examination of the Craze, see Phillips, supra, 123–131 and Gately, supra, 159–174.

[134] Phillips, supra, 126.

Reflecting this belief, William Hogarth's famous etching, "Gin Lane" (1751), illustrates a disheveled nursing mother so inebriated that she fails to notice that her infant has slipped away and is falling into the street. Is Hogarth's etching evidence? It is, at least, reflective of a widespread public belief. Yet in support of that belief, others made substantive (if not substantiated) claims, e.g., that gin-drinking reduced the appetite for nutritious food, led to crime, and disrupted family stability. For example, a tract from 1736 entitled *The trial of spirits: or, some considerations upon the pernicious consequences of the gin-trade to Great Britain (as it is Destructive of the Health and Lives of His Majesty's Subjects…)* cites "the most enormous, wicked and dangerous *Use* and *Consequences* of the Liquor call'd Gin or Genevra" (2). During the period covered by the Eighteenth Century Collection Online, 53,620 separate works commented on gin; if you rank them according to "relevance," virtually all the first several that we examined are highly critical.

So, while "gin craze" is an ambidextrous phrase (suggesting that the public was crazed, perhaps as much or more than gin's consumers), the sheer accessibility of gin was probably responsible for creating one of the earliest episodes of unrestrained drinking accompanied by a massive public outcry against it. In 1736 and 1751, Parliament passed a series of Gin Acts aimed at reducing the prevalence of gin and its perceived negative impacts on society.

But distilled spirits were hardly confined to Europe.

As the Dutch, British, and French expanded their settlements in the Americas, they exported their knowledge of distilling (along with religion and diseases). Settler economies applied this knowledge to make their own distilled spirits, which they exported back to Europe. Notoriously, this was the case of rum, which played a crucial role in the so-called Triangular Trade (16th through 19th centuries) involving Europe, Africa, and the Americas. In a rough outline, rum, produced in New England from molasses, was traded for manufactures and other goods from Europe, which were then traded for slaves from Africa. The slaves were then transported to the West Indies to work on sugar plantations, where molasses was made from sugar to make rum, perpetuating the cycle.[135] In the late 18th century, some British consumers were so horrified by the sugar/slavery connection that they boycotted sugar, even while (in a split-screen vision of reality) cookbooks promoted the confectioner's art.[136]

In the early 18th century, France banned the distillation of rum in its West Indian colonies to deter competition with brandy made domestically. This, however, allowed New England distillers to undersell their British West Indian competitors by buying reduced-price molasses from French plantations. When British rum producers predictably became incensed, they persuaded Parliament to pass the Molasses Act of 1733, taxing molasses imports into Britain's American colonies from foreign countries or colonies. Since paying the duty would have made further production too expensive, the Americans largely failed to comply. The Act was followed by the Sugar Act of 1764, which, like the infamous Stamp Act, may have been in the drafters' minds when the Declaration of Independence blamed King George III for assenting to laws that "impos[e] Taxes on us without Consent."

Yet cheap molasses could not survive the Revolutionary War. Imports dried up; the rum industry took a hit. Nor could

---

[135] The triangular trade has been exhaustively studied. See, e.g., Emert PR (ed.). (2010) *Colonial Triangular Trade: An Economy Based on Human Misery*. Applewood Books. Though many routes varied and trade patterns were more complex, the role of rum remained critical.

[136] See Sherman, supra, *Invention of the Modern Cookbook*.

the industry easily bounce back. Moreover, the emancipation of 750,000 West Indian slaves (1834), plus depleted soil, threw sugar production into a decline. As a result, sugar (and molasses) became more expensive. There was an opening for whiskey. Given the endless expanses of grain (no one fretted about shortages), growth in the distillation of bourbon, rye, and other whiskeys was foreordained. But just like the British with gin, the post-war U.S. government sought to profit off whiskey and, thereby, cover debts it had incurred in fighting the British. In 1791, it imposed a whiskey tax, with a graduated rate that nonetheless affected small producers disproportionately. The result was the Whiskey Rebellion, a series of violent eruptions that only subsided when troops led by George Washington finally put them down.[137] But continued enforcement of the tax was weak, and it was abolished in 1802. As Cockx drily observes, "Discussions over whiskey regulations switched from raising tax revenue to restricting excess consumption."[138]

Of course, the Whiskey Rebellion was never really defeated; it just adopted other means. The Distilled Spirits Council, along with individual spirits producers, spends millions annually on lobbying. On its website, it claims to seek increased market access for consumers by opposing high state taxes — a potential contradiction to its other stated goal of promoting responsible consumption. In a response to the 2025 Advisory by the U.S. Surgeon General that linked even moderate alcohol consumption to the risk of cancer,[139] the Council suggested that the Advisory had missed the wider

---

[137] The Rebellion was an early test of government authority. For a detailed discussion of the politics, see *Killer High*, supra, 29–36.

[138] Cockx, supra, at 13.

[139] The report is at https://www.hhs.gov/surgeongeneral/reports-and-publications/alcohol-cancer/index.html.

picture.[140] What the Rebellion and its long aftermath demonstrate, is that distilled spirits are embedded in the politics of how taxes are levied and how health is discussed. It has been that way at least since the Gin Craze.

Whiskey was also produced by the Scots and Irish, first in the monasteries and then, when they were closed by Henry VIII, by households and farms (mainly for their own consumption). Not long after, commercial distillers saw an opportunity. Demand was growing, domestically and in the British Empire. Whiskey was an important export, with consequences that have been well-documented.[141] Yet whiskey was not one product; it varied according to where it was produced. In the Scottish Highlands, it was distilled from malted barley; in the Lowlands, it was made from grain, where it might also be "blended" from various products to create a more consistent taste. But nothing was ever tranquil regarding whiskey. As Cockx observes:

> The history of whisky in Scotland and Ireland is also a history of taxes, regulations, and evasion. In times of poor grain harvests, the government tried to ban whisky distilling. When budgets were needed to finance wars, the government raised taxes on whisky. One of the most well-known taxes was the Malt Tax introduced in Britain in 1725, which caused much upheaval among whisky producers. However, as with all whisky regulations and taxes, small distillers in the northern Scottish Highlands were better positioned

[140] See https://www.distilledspirits.org/news/discus-statement-in-response-to-surgeon-generals-advisory/#:~:text=Statement%20Attributed%20to%20Dr., not%20review%20broader%20health%20outcomes

[141] See, e.g., Burton KD. (2015) Intoxication and empire: Distilled spirits and the creation of addiction in the early Modern British Atlantic.

to evade whisky taxes and regulations than the larger and registered distilleries in the Lowlands. This resulted in substantial smuggling of illegal whisky from the Highlands to the southern regions.[142]

Whiskey smuggling had a long, glorious history in Scotland.[143] It was another outcropping of the smuggler's trade that flourished in Britain for centuries, involving an array of commodities, such as tea, silk, and brandy.[144] Primarily, it was motivated by economics, but (among some Scots) there was also a cultural element grounded in defiance of authority (that is, a *foreign* authority, as England was considered to be among those who never accepted the Act of Union [1707]). Smuggling was never entirely stamped out.

As consumption of distilled spirits grew in the 19th century, they were stigmatized as unnatural, and thus to be avoided (unlike wine and beer, which were said to be harmless — even healthful — if consumed in moderation). The claim, which rejected any degree of "temperance" when it came to spirits, made the case that while wine and beer were made by small wineries and brewers, who barely intervened in nature, spirits were made in large, industrial facilities that used complicated equipment. Clearly, the claim did

---

[142] Cockx, 14.

[143] White S. (2020) *Smugglers and Excisemen: The History of Whisky in Scotland, 1644 to 1823*. Master's thesis, The University of Western Ontario, Canada.

[144] See Rosenberger B. (2020) The British smuggling dilemma: 1698–1784. *Int ResearchScape J* **7**(1), 5; Monod P. (1991) Dangerous merchandise: Smuggling, Jacobitism, and commercial culture in Southeast England, 1690–1760. *J Brit Stud* **30**(2), 150–182; Ramsay GD (1952) The smugglers' trade: A neglected aspect of English commercial development. *Trans R Hist Soc* **2**, 131–157.

not reflect reality: there were thousands of small stills all over the U.S. and Europe, and beer was produced by huge London brewers. Nonetheless, it sublimated a growing alarm in "polite" society regarding the effect of industrialization, which drew masses of working-class people to the cities where they got publicly drunk (unlike wealthier people, who could hide their excesses at home or in private clubs). Apparently, however, the working classes were not concerned with what we would call "wellness." In Britian, consumption of spirits almost doubled from 1826 to 1830.[145] From 1824 to 1874, the population grew by 88%, while sales of spirits distilled grew by 237% and sales of spirits produced outside Britain grew by 152%.[146] These sales were helped, in part, by the shortage of wine imports from France, where the phylloxera (a tiny insect) had attacked vines and almost wiped out the entire wine-making industry.

Because of the shortage, wine-drinkers in France also turned to distilled spirits, though they also developed a heightened interest in beer, which had always been considered quintessentially British. Still, between 1870 and 1890, French production of distilled spirits doubled.[147] One spirit that gripped the French imagination was absinthe, originally introduced into France in 1840, and popularized in the 1960s and 70s.[148] It was green and mysterious,

---

[145] Phillips, 176.

[146] Phillps, 177. The statistics regarding liquor consumption are so precise because, starting in the late 18th century, quantification had become the norm in all areas of public life. See Sherman, *Imagining Poverty*, supra.

[147] Phillips, 179.

[148] Absinthe is certainly irresistible to historians. See, e.g., Bresseur T, *et al.* (2024) *Absinth — The Forbidden Spirit: An Intoxicating History of the Green Fairy*. Helvetiq; Wittels B & Breaux TA. (2017) *Absinthe: The Exquisite Elixir.*

distilled from wormwood, and consumed conspicuously by an avant-garde of Parisian aesthetes — Pail Verlaine, Henri Toulouse Lautrec, Vincent van Gogh, Edgar Degas. It was associated with decadence. It was 40% alcohol (wine was <1/3 of that), possibly hallucinatory, and it made you drunk fast. Phillips observes that "it was the first alcoholic beverage to be banned outright in many countries."[149] The campaign to prohibit it was galvanized when a peasant, drunk on absinthe, murdered his pregnant wife and two daughters because the wife had failed to wax his boots.

Absinthe is available in most liquor stores. In New York City, specialty absinthe bars have names like Café L'enfer (translation: Café Hell), Please Don't Tell, and Oscar Wilde (alluding to the high priest of decadence). Some things never change.

Americans' consumption of whiskey increased when imports of molasses for making rum ceased during the Revolutionary War. Whiskey was blamed for crime, poverty, and domestic violence. Employers complained that employees arrived at work drunk. But whiskey-drinking was encouraged in the American army, where soldiers received a daily ration of whiskey; only in 1832 was that replaced by coffee or tea, following repeated reports of drunkenness and even desertion. Washington, who was always sober, had five corn stills at Mount Vernon. During the Civil War, General Ulysses S. Grant was famous for drinking Old Crow bourbon. You can still buy Old Crow Kentucky Straight Bourbon Whiskey, which, in a sense, is a direct link to the hard-drinking tradition of the American army.

Chicago Review Press — Fulcrum; Conrad B. (1997) *Absinthe: History in a Bottle*. Chronicle Books.

[149] Id.

Chapter 4 – Tobacco

Archaeological evidence points to the use of tobacco as early as the mid-11th century B.C.E.[150] The evidence consists of four charred *Nicotiana* seeds found at a hearth site in the Great Salt Lake Desert in northern Utah.[151] The find is astonishing because it antedates the prior demonstrated use of tobacco by 9000 years! Still, how could seeds, which are not smoked and contain no nicotine, indicate the use of tobacco as a stimulant? After determining that the seeds probably didn't come from the remains of ducks cooked at the site, or that they weren't simply used as fuel, the archaeologists explain how the seeds could have hitched a ride during a range of activities using the *leaves*:

> The data suggest use [of tobacco] as a fireside activity along with food preparation, consumption, and tool use among mobile-hunter-gatherers at distance from natural tobacco habitat. The finding of seeds implies emphasis on leaves and flowering stems, the parts with the intoxicant effect. Seeds are the tobacco parts preserved most often in the archaeobotanical record, but non-germinated seeds carry no nicotine. Because seeds are small and easily caught up by the sticky hairs of the plant, they could be incidentally included when leaves and stems with attached flowering parts are

---

[150] Duke D, Wohlgemuth E, Adams K, *et al.* (2022). Earliest evidence for human use of tobacco in Pleistocene America. *Nat Hum Behav* **6**, 183–192. See also, Nuwer R. (2021) Mammoths roamed when humans started using tobacco at least 12,300 years ago. *Sci Am*, https://www.scientificamerican.com/article/mammoths-roamed-when-humans-started-using-tobacco-at-least-12-300-years-ago/

[151] Dating relied on three radiocarbon age estimates of pieces of charred willow from the hearth fill.

harvested. This is consistent with the archaeological record and preparation methods by native groups in the Great Basin.[152]

So, if these Paleolithic humans sat around the fire high on nicotine, how did they consume it? Evidence from precontact pipes suggests that smoking was common — the seeds might have been left behind as "unused portions of undesired dry remains."[153] But chewing wads and sucking quids were also common; seeds (found in 90% of quids examined at an Arizona site) might have been spat into the fire, while expended quids might have just been tossed in.

The find has implications for humans' early relationship with intoxicating plants, which, in the case of *Nicotiana*, were growing in the wild. It also sheds light on the lengthy (though likely discontinuous) cultural experience with tobacco that led to its domestication, thousands of years later, among people who by then were sedentary. What the find does not reveal is how these Paleolithic people first discovered nicotine's intoxicating properties. In this regard, we can only speculate, as we must with coca and opium.

Yet, while we can now resituate humans' first encounter with tobacco, there is new evidence that tobacco was also smoked over 3200 years ago among indigenous peoples in western U.S., who had been thought to be ignorant of it until Euro-American traders offered it to them in the late 18th century.[154] This new evidence helps connect the dots in establishing tobacco's trajectory from

---

[152] See prepublication version of "Earliest evidence of human use of tobacco," supra, https://assets-eu.researchsquare.com/files/rs-139445/v1_covered.pdf?c=1637595171, ll. 153–162.

[153] Id. ll. 165–166.

[154] See Tushingham S, Snyder CM, Brownstein KJ, *et al.* (2018) Biomolecular archaeology reveals ancient origins of indigenous tobacco smoking in North American Plateau. *Proc Nat Acad Sci* **115**(46), 11742–11747.

wild plant to domestication. Additionally, and looking back towards the earliest uses of tobacco, the study makes a more general, historiographical observation that "the spread of domesticated trade tobacco seems to have overtaken and obscured indigenous tobacco practices."[155] In other words, any history of tobacco use by indigenous people should not make assumptions whereby the fact of conquest obscures how and whether such people used tobacco prior to contact with Euro-Americans. This approach would align with trends in social science to move beyond Western-centered perspectives by recognizing the agency of people being studied.

Tushingham and collaborators demonstrate that at five sites in the Columbia River Basin in (what is now) southeast Washington State, hunter-gatherer communities, including ancient Nez Perce peoples, smoked wild tobacco well before domesticated tobacco was introduced by Euro-American fur traders and settlers after 1790. The evidence consists of pipes and pipe fragments containing tobacco biomarkers. It establishes that tobacco was smoked in areas vastly distant from South America and the Caribbean, where tobacco was also smoked even earlier, but which had not been in contact with the North American west coast.

Ancient, indigenous peoples in the southern hemisphere had used tobacco for millennia.[156] According to plant geneticists studying tobacco remains, humans were growing tobacco in the Peruvian/Ecuadorian highlands as early as 5000–3000 B.C.E.[157]

---

[155] Id.

[156] Though tobacco emerged in western South America, the plant moved north via Central America, then across the southern U.S. to the west.

[157] Gilman SL & Zhou X (eds.). (2004) *Smoke: A Global History of Smoking*. Reaktion Books, 9; Gately I. (2007) *Tobacco: A Cultural History of How an Exotic Plant Seduced Civilization*. Open Road+ Grove/Atlantic, 3.

This is only a millennium or so later than the first documented use of coca in the same region. Like coca, tobacco was used to reward warriors; it had religious and medicinal significance and was also used to suppress appetite during times of stress. But unlike coca, it provided no extended stimulation; rather, it caused a quick, temporary release of adrenaline and endorphins that — as the Europeans discovered — led to addiction when the user sought to remain "high." The drugs were also consumed differently. Coca was chewed; tobacco was inhaled, a more efficient means of conveying its psychoactive molecule (nicotine) to the brain. Yet as Iain Gately observes, the means of tobacco consumption still varied:

> Tobacco was sniffed, chewed, eaten, drunk, smeared over bodies, used in eye drops and enemas, and smoked. It was blown into warriors' faces before battle, over fields before planting and over women prior to sex, it was offered to the gods, and accepted as their gift, and not least it served as a simple narcotic for daily use by men and women.[158]

These uses, embedded with shamanistic cultural practices, carried associations to fertility, medication, and war.[159] Though, like coca, tobacco could be used daily, where addictive behaviors (as we define them) were likely controlled by limiting access to

---

[158] Gately, Tobacco, 5. The plant originated in South America around 65 million years ago. See Sadik T. (2014) Traditional use of tobacco among indigenous peoples in North America, in *Chippewas of the Thames First Nation*.

[159] See Chapter 2, Food of the Spirits: Shamanism, healing and tobacco in Amerindian culture, in Goodman J. (2005) *Tobacco in History: The Cultures of Dependence*. Routledge. Goodman observes that "Amerindian societies located tobacco within a specific cosmology of which the art of healing was a critical component," 37.

specific individuals for specific purposes, who used the drug in limited quantities. Indigenous traditions involved respectful use, not habitual or recreational use in the modern sense.

Still, one scholar cites accounts dating back to the 16th century that describe a heavy dependence on tobacco among North American indigenous populations.[160] The problem is that in interpreting these accounts from a Western, secular perspective, we risk creating a false dichotomy between "addiction" and traditional, sacred practices requiring tobacco use.[161] Of course, this sacredness was compromised when, late in the 18th century, indigenous populations began trading fur for southern-grown tobacco offered by Euro-Americans.[162] By then, tobacco was a commodity.

Ironically, an Englishman, Thomas Hariot, became one of the first known addicts. Hariot, a respected researcher, accompanied the first English colonists to Roanoke Island in 1585, and reported that he and many others "used to sucke [tobacco] after [the Amerindian] manner, as also since our returne." But such use was only superficially like the indigenes': it was habitual rather than medicinal. Hariot died of cancer of the nose, apparently caused by exhaling tobacco smoke along the nasal passageways.[163] In 1610, Francis Bacon wrote what is believed to be the first

---

[160] See Von Gernet A. (2000) North American indigenous *Nicotiana* use and tobacco shamanism: The early documentary record: 1520–1660, in *Tobacco Use by Native North Americans: Sacred Smoke and Silent Killer*, Vol. 236, Winter JC (ed.). University of Oklahoma Press.

[161] Sadik, 7. See Sadik for an extensive review of tobacco use in religious practices among indigenous peoples (including the Aztec) across North America.

[162] Cured tobacco was traded for furs even though it was also derived from a local plant. Because the tobacco was southern-grown, it was produced by slaves.

[163] Goodman observes "that Hariot became addicted to tobacco . . . is well established," 48.

written account of tobacco addiction: "Tobacco conquers men with a secret pleasure, so that those who have once become accustomed thereto can later hardly be restrained therefrom."[164]

Tobacco penetrated Europe more quickly than coca because, unlike coca, the dried, cured leaves are good travelers. By the 17th century, Virginia was exporting ~380,000 pounds of tobacco a year to England.[165] In effect, the tobacco trade went in two directions: from the Americas to Europe, and from Virginia and the Caribbean to points across the North American continent.

The story of tobacco's arrival in Europe followed a path similar to coca's. Some members of Columbus' crew acquired the habit.[166] The Spanish conquest of the Americas helped spread the drug throughout Europe.[167] Tobacco existed in England at least since the 1560s, when sailors returning from a voyage captained by Merchant Adventurer Sir John Hawkins brought it with them. They likely picked up the habit from Spanish and Portuguese sailors.[168] British wars in Europe spread the habit; Dutch armies acquired the habit from the English and spread it even further. The French practice of inhaling tobacco (taking "snuff") followed

---

[164] See Sanchez-Ramos JR. (2020) The rise and fall of tobacco as a botanical medicine. *J Herb Med* **22**, 100374.

[165] Goodman, 59.

[166] Andreas, supra, 69.

[167] In 1570, King Philip II of Spain commissioned an expedition to bring back information on medicinal plants native to Mexico. Over a period of years, the expedition leader, Francisco Hernandez de Toledo, "collected and described over 3000 plants." See Goodman, 38.

[168] See https://www.nationalarchives.gov.uk/education/resources/tobacco/. Sir Walter Raleigh is sometimes credited with introducing tobacco to England, but this notion is questionable.

its introduction by the diplomat, Jean Nicot, whose name is immortalized in nicotine.

In late Tudor England, courtiers took up tobacco as a symbol of their colonial ambitions (as in the hit movie, *Shakespeare in Love* [1998], where Lord Wessex will found a tobacco plantation in Virginia).[169] At the time, most tobacco consumed in Europe was sourced from Spain, where the climate was well-suited to its cultivation. The French were also growers, but the plant originated in the Americas, where the English had yet to develop a colony (by 1590, the Roanoke Colony had failed). The Stuarts finally realized Tudor ambitions with the establishment of Jamestown.

By the late 16th century, tobacco had spread to Japan, and the shogun tried to ban it. But he failed, and tobacco was legalized in 1625.[170] Samurai carried ornate silver pipes for smoking it.[171] The Japanese, who occupied the Korean peninsula, likely introduced it to Korea and Manchuria. In the 17th century, smoking also spread to Persia, despite fierce initial opposition from Shah Abbas I.

Back in England, King James I asked the obvious question: was the habit of any value? James hated tobacco. In the early 17th century, it was still essentially Spanish and, hence, associated with the Catholic church (James was raised Presbyterian, and leaned Anglican).[172] In his *Countrblaste to Tobacco* (1604), considered the

---

[169] Harley D. (1993) The beginnings of the tobacco controversy: Puritanism, James I, and the Royal Physicians. *Bull Hist Med* **67**, 26–50.

[170] The shogun's attempt is an uncanny anticipation of failed Chinese attempts to ban opium.

[171] Andreas, 71.

[172] James' mother, Queen Mary of Scots ("Bloody Mary") had tried to restore Catholicism in England. On the complex religious — and, hence, political — issues surrounding tobacco in the late 17th and early 18th centuries, see Harley, supra.

earliest significant opposition to the drug,[173] James depicts smoking as an existential threat, a symptom of brewing national decline:

> Our Peace hath bred wealth: and Peace and wealth hath brought foorth a general sluggishnesse, which makes us wallow in all sorts of idle delights and soft delicacies, the first seedes of the subversion of all great Monarchies.[174]

James' language evokes decadence, even emasculation: an idle, wallowing, "sluggishnesse." It is the opposite of what, a century later, was seen as Britain's hypermasculine advantage over France — beer. Tobacco consumption poses a political threat ("the first seedes of… subversion") which, as a new king and a Scot, James might have feared. The *Counterblastehe* also raised aesthetic objections (tobacco stinks) and observed that smoking harmed the brain, nose, and lungs. Not surprisingly, he raised the tax on tobacco from 2 p to 82 p per pound, before it fell back and stabilized at 24 p by 1615.

But English subjects kept consuming the drug. James bowed to reality. In an about-face, he created a royal monopoly on the trade in 1624, which, in effect, capitalized on tobacco's popularity. Profits went directly to the Crown,[175] setting a precedent for British governments to continue deriving revenue from the trade.

---

[173] There was an earlier, less prominent outburst against the drug. In 1602, a pamphlet entitled *Work for Chimny-Sweepers or a Warning for Tabbaccanists*, by a physician calling himself Philaretes, claimed that tobacco was a poison, and that its use deprived the body of nourishment, diminished men's sperm, and had a stupefying effect much like opium's. The cover contained the motto: "Better chok't with English hemp, then poisoned with Indian Tobacco."

[174] *Countrblaste*, Preface.

[175] See New York Public Library web page on the *Counterblaste*, https://www.nypl.org/events/exhibitions/galleries/beginnings/item/3556

Yet apart from the fact that people liked tobacco, did James' opposition ever stand a chance? Probably not. It would have interfered with access to an established medical treatment. Travelers starting with Columbus brought back stories of its use by indigenous peoples to cure a range of ailments.[176] In the 17th century, most herbs were thought to have beneficial effects when used appropriately. Beautifully illustrated herbals overflowed with such advice. During this relatively early stage of tobacco's reception in the West, it too was assumed to have (and was, lauded for) medicinal properties.[177] In 1618, the Royal College of Physicians issued the *Pharmacopoeia Londinensis*, recommending hot, dry tobacco as a cure for colds and lethargy.[178] It was used to treat a variety of ailments from earaches to asthma and syphilis. Later in the century, as physicians began observing the effects of tobacco,

---

[176] Charlton A. (2004) Medical uses of tobacco in history. *J R Soc Med* **97**, 292–296. On the medicinal use of tobacco by indigenous peoples, and subsequent medical applications in the West, see Charlton; Stewart GG. (1967) A history of the medicinal use of tobacco 1492–1860. *Med Hist* **11**(3), 228–268; Sanchez-Ramos, supra; and Goodman, supra.

[177] Goodman observes that during the 16th century, tobacco "was becoming accepted as a herbal therapy capable of curing an increasingly large number of ailments. Under the scrutiny of a host of European botanists, physicians, churchmen and bureaucrats… tobacco picked up one accolade after another," 44.

[178] Early Modern medicine, still in thrall to Galenic, humoral doctrines ("hot," "cold," "wet," "dry"), regarded tobacco as "hot" and "dry" — physicians prescribed it to rebalance the humors of someone seen as cold. The *Pharmacopoeia* probably drew on work by Nicolas Monardes (1571), the prominent Seville physician who established tobacco's humoral essence — hot and dry — and cited more than 20 ailments that tobacco cured. It may also have been influenced by Giles Everard's *De herba panacea* (1587), which collected an array of Galenic uses for tobacco. James' *Counterblaste* felt compelled to debate tobacco's supposed humoral virtues.

opposition developed,[179] but tobacco continued to be used medicinally through the 19th century.

Snuff-taking (the inhalation of powdered tobacco often mixed with sweet herbs)[180], became hugely popular, and finally overtook smoking — to the detriment of pipe manufacturers, and the benefit of craftsmen who specialized in snuff boxes.[181] It became a status-marker. The higher classes considered it a daintier, more elegant form of consuming tobacco (pipes were for everyone else).

Yet taking snuff could just as easily tip into over-refinement, as in late 17th-century Restoration Comedy, where dandified characters ("fops") were portrayed as avid snuff-takers.[182] Incongruously, snuff caused sneezing. In the heroine's Epilogue to *The Bath, or the Western Lass* (1701), playwright Thomas D'Urfey winks at an audience, likely to ridicule snuff even while taking it themselves:

---

[179] In 1620, for example, Thomas Venner's *Via Recta* argued that overuse of tobacco degraded the eyes, harmed the brain, interfered with digestion, and induced trembling. Simon Pauli's *Commentarius de Abusu Tabaci*... (1661) advocated tobacco's destruction. On the increasing opposition to tobacco, see Sanchez-Ramos, supra. Compare the 17th-century trajectory of sugar, which, early in the century, was sometimes used in balancing the humors — until later, when physicians noticed its negative effects, e.g., on teeth.

[180] As a "flavored" alternative to smoking, snuff-taking has uncanny similarities to vaping. In 1493, a Catholic monk who accompanied Columbus on this second voyage to the West Indies gave an extensive description of snuff-taking among the indigenes. See Russo P, *et al.* (2011) Tobacco habit: Historical, cultural, neurobiological, and genetic features of people's relationship with an addictive drug, *Perspect Biol Med* **54**(4), 557–577, 561.

[181] Goodman cites an "unmistakable decline" in British pipe-makers, especially after the middle of the 18th century, 71.

[182] See Ramczyk S. (2002). *Delicious Dissembling: A Complete Guide to Performing Restoration Comedy* (Heinemann Drama), which examines the etiquette of period necessities like bowing, using a fan, and taking snuff.

Now that th'Opera's gaudy Scenes have shown the show
And the Beauties of May-Fair are vanish'd too,
I hope I may appear in *Statu quo*,
For I must own, whilst the Rope dancing sway'd,
I did take snuff, you should my Face degrade;
Gad, I began to think my charms decay'd.

Women took snuff. An ever-larger swath of the male population took it. Benjamin Franklin accepted a diamond-encrusted snuff box from Louis XVI. Napoleon collected snuff boxes.

Even if you weren't rich, snuff-taking allowed you (if only in a small way) to imagine yourself as richer. You could splurge on making your own mixtures, adding a variety of herbs and fragrances (e.g., mint, bergamot, cloves, spirit of oranges). You could buy fine-sounding mixtures prepared by tobacconists. Snuff was not just everyday tobacco; rather, it was the culmination of a complex, artisanal process that transformed tobacco. Goodman observes that it "required an elaborate operation of moistening with the liquor containing the flavourings, colours and essences and consecutive drying processes taking at least three weeks before it was ready."[183] All the reek of tobacco — which infuriated James — was strained away. What remained was literally refined, and it reflected on you.

Snuff boxes made statements on their own. As Goodman remarks, the boxes were "the equivalent of jewellery," so that "not only did the snuff box change with artistic fashion but anyone who was anyone needed to have a variety of these boxes."[184] They could be expertly crafted of precious materials — Marie Antoinette

[183] Goodman, 74.

[184] Goodman, 74.

received 52 gold boxes ahead of her marriage to Louis XVI. In a brilliant article, Vanessa Alayrac-Fielding analyzes how snuff boxes could normalize and aestheticize the slave system that made possible a large portion of tobacco production.[185]

Yet apart from any status that snuff and its paraphernalia conferred — or, at least, allowed you to imagine — there were other grounds for consuming it: snuff was said to be less damaging to internal organs than pipe-smoking; it was even said to be healthful in that, for example, sneezing expelled "corrupt humors."[186] In any case, you didn't have to carry a flint, since snuff required no spark (so you wouldn't risk burning yourself).

But despite the ostensible benefits, the downside of snuff was that *it was still tobacco*. In 1761, the British physician John Hill published *Cautions against the Immoderate Use of Snuff*, which may have been the earliest clinical study of tobacco's effects.[187] The treatise begins brutally:

> Tobacco is a narcotic with a peculiar acrimony.
> 'Tis such a body as art might prepare might mixing Opium with Euphorbium.
> The herb itself is so nearly poisonous, that no physician gives it inwardly. (4)

---

[185] Alayrac-Fielding V. (2021) From Oroonoko tobacco to blackamoor snuff-boxes: Race, gender and the consumption of snuff in eighteenth-century Britain. *Humanities* **10**(3), 92.

[186] In the sense that taking snuff was said to mitigate the damage posed by smoking, it anticipated claims made by filter cigarettes over three centuries later. On the supposed benefits attributed to snuff, see Goodman, 78–80.

[187] See Russo, supra.

Hill then becomes graphic, describing the delicate nasal passages and snuff's effect on them: "[P]ersons accustomed to Snuff, no longer sneeze on taking it. The powder, which was at first thrown off so violently, is permitted to lodge, and to exert all its force. The Nerves are thus corroded and destroyed, and the sense of smelling, is impaired; and, in the end, totally lost" (10). If anyone thought snuff was glamorous, Hill was out to disabuse them. He does for snuff what the Atlantic slave trade did for the rise of tobacco. In both instances, the dark side of tobacco (and tobacco products) obliterates whatever pleasure tobacco may afford.

Commerce in tobacco was a phenomenon of the Atlantic world and was a driving force in the trans-Atlantic history of slavery. In 1612, John Rolfe successfully grew the Virginia colony's first tobacco crop, using seeds from Trinidad. Over the next 160 years, production spread from the Tidewater area to the Blue Ridge Mountains. It dominated the agriculture of the Chesapeake region (i.e., Virginia and Maryland).[188] Income from tobacco was used to buy slaves and indentured servants, pay taxes, and purchase manufactures from England. By 1700, the Chesapeake was exporting over 37 million pounds of tobacco a year to England; by 1771, that figure was over 100 million pounds.[189] Slaves outnumbered indentured servants (who worked off the price of their passage) and, as employment opportunities in England improved, planters made up for the loss in workers by buying more slaves. As Goodman observes, the introduction of slaves altered the region's fundamental social structure:

---

[188] See Salmon E & Salmon J. (2020) Tobacco in colonial Virginia, in *Encyclopedia Virginia*, https://encyclopediavirginia.org/entries/tobacco-in-colonial-virginia/

[189] Goodman, 146.

> Beginning in the 1680s and then accelerating at a fantastic rate, Chesapeake society was transformed from a society based on [indentured] servitude to one based on slavery; from relative egalitarian to rigidly hierarchical; and from ethnically European to ethnically African.[190]

Whereas blacks comprised only 13% of the population in 1700, that figure was 40% by 1780.[191] Between 1698 and 1774, ~80,000–100,000 slaves arrived in Virginia.[192] The PBS series *Jamestown* (2016–2018), dramatizes the early history of tobacco-planting in the region (primarily 1619–1622), depicting the arrival of slaves and the brutality of slavery as an institution.

Impressed by tobacco's success, European powers planted it in their own Caribbean and South American colonies. Brazil, with its vast expanses, became an export powerhouse and a major supplier to Britain. Nearly 2 million Africans were transported to Brazil between 1700 and 1800, on top of 560,000 between 1650 and 1700. Goodman observes that "As for the Americas, it was slavery as an institution and the slave trade as a capitalist enterprise that shaped the nature of tobacco societies until the middle of the nineteenth century…"[193]

During the 17th and 18th centuries, tobacco prices fluctuated due to wars in Europe (which disrupted British shipping), the unstable British economy, and over-production at home. By the 1770s, most planters, who traded on credit, were heavily in debt.

---

[190] Id., 176.

[191] Id.

[192] Salmon & Salmon, supra. Most slaves in colonial Virginia worked on tobacco, not cotton plantations. While cotton was a significant crop in the South, it was not the primary crop in Virginia during this period.

[193] Goodman, 189.

When British banks collapsed in 1772 and pressured planters to settle their accounts, the ensuing credit crisis may have helped push the planters toward revolution.[194] At the very least, they could have escaped the so-called mercantile system (in which the Crown sets prices), which required all shipments to use British vessels and prohibited trade with third countries.[195] By the time of the Revolution, tobacco exporters were paying duties of £300,000 to the Crown.[196] After the war, tobacco exports helped pay off the war debt.[197] There was mounting awareness of slavery's toll, but not enough to dislodge it.

Perhaps the most interesting development of the period was the Americans adopting the cigar as a patriotic statement, to distinguish themselves from the pipe-smoking British.[198] Cigar-smoking further increased after the Mexican-American War (1846–1848), when the Americans observed the enemy smoking them, a habit picked up from the Spanish. Mark Twain was virtually never without a cigar and was handsomely paid to advertise them. His doctors warned him that smoking was slowly killing him (he had chronic bronchitis and a heart condition), but Twain remained happily addicted.

---

[194] Breen TH. (2001) *Tobacco Culture: The Mentality of the Great Tidewater Planters on the Eve of Revolution*. Princeton University Press. George Washington, Thomas Jefferson, and Patrick Henry — all tobacco growers — resented the system.

[195] In *Common Sense* (1776), Tom Paine opposed the mercantile system, arguing that the colonies would be better off if they untethered to Britain.

[196] Andreas, 70.

[197] Andreas, 73.

[198] Andreas, 74. Cigars first arrived in America through an officer who picked up the habit (where else?) in Cuba during the Seven Years War (1756–1763).

In the early 20th century, cigars' popularity began to decline, as cigarettes gained in popularity.[199] By then, of course, any patriotic associations with cigars had long vanished. But ironically, British soldiers fighting Napoleon in the early 19th century took up cigars when their snuff boxes proved unwieldy. For both the British and Americans, cigars thus served as cigarettes-on-training-wheels, weaning them away from forms of tobacco that required paraphernalia like pipes, pipe-cleaners, tobacco pouches, and snuff-boxes. In Britain, such "training" bore quick results. The first cigarette factory opened in Britain in 1856. Then Philip Morris, a London tobacconist selling pipe tobacco and cigars, introduced cigarette brands named after Britain's elite universities, Oxford and Cambridge. When Americans visiting Britain encountered cigarettes, they could have brought them home.

But it took a while for cigarettes to displace cigars (and pipes, chewing tobacco, and snuff). During the Civil War, Ulysses S. Grant smoked cigars, and leaf tobacco was part of men's rations on both sides. For a while, soldiers smoked cigarettes because they were easily portable, but they returned to their former cigar/pipe/snuff habits once the war ended. Pipes and cigars were considered

---

[199] For a chart tracing cigars' popularity and subsequent decline, see Burns DM. (1998) Cigar smoking: Overview and current state of the science. *Smoking and Tobacco Control Monograph* **9**, 1–19. Cigars later made a slight comeback in the 1950s and 60s as the dangers of cigarette-smoking were publicized. More recently, cigar events and the emergence of cigar bars have also added to their popularity. See Gerlach KK, Cummings KM, Hyland A, *et al.* (1998) Trends in cigar consumption and smoking prevalence, in *National Cancer Institute, Cigars. Health Effects and Trends*, 21–52. On the growing popularity of cigars among women, see Female cigar smoking — A growing trend, https://sigars.com/blog/female-cigar-smokers-a-growing-trend#:~:text=Cigar%20smoking%20has%20long%20been,cigars%20gain%20popularity%20among%20women

the more masculine smoke; cigarettes had associations with the decadent Spanish. It took the First World War to finally — and irrevocably — tip the balance. During the war, military leaders encouraged smoking to maintain morale, maintain alertness, and suppress hunger.[200] As Andreas remarks, "[A]t the end of the war, almost all of the returning American soldiers brought their cigarette habit back with them. Unlike the years after the Civil War, this time the habit stuck. Cigarette use by soldiers and civilians alike surged."[201] As more women entered the workplace during and after the war, they picked up the habit as well.

Women smoking

Yet World War I did not even start until 1914, when cigarettes had already made some inroads on cigars. Therefore, by situating the cigar-to-cigarette paradigm shift in the years just following the war, we exclude developments in the 50+ years after the Civil War and before World War I. In fact, as it turns out, however much *soldiers* accustomed themselves to cigarettes during World War I, and however much women in the workforce emulated them, women's adoption of cigarettes in the years preceding World War I was a separate trajectory that did not just track the men's. Moreover, to the extent that women's own experience set in motion distinctive post-war patterns — say, in advertising cigarettes directly to women — those patterns should also be considered, even though they finally converge with wartime and post-war developments that involved men.

During the 19th century, when cigarettes were emerging but cigars still predominated, when and how did women begin

---

[200] Andreas, 81.

[201] Andreas, 80–81.

smoking? Some smoked cigars in private; some smoked them in public as a sign of nonconformity. The more interesting story, however, is how women were *depicted* smoking cigarettes.[202] A promotional shot (1851) of "Lola Montez, the Spanish Dancer" is one of the earliest photos of anyone holding a cigarette. As Amanda Amos and Margarethe Haglund observe, the cigarette was "used as a focal point of the picture," and "was intended to be provocative."[203] Montez made her Broadway debut in 1851, preceded by notoriety. George Bizet's opera, *Carmen*, features a Spanish heroine who works in a cigarette factory, smokes cigarettes, and seduces men. First staged in New York City in 1878, "it helped reinforce the American image of cigarette smoking as exotically foreign and sinful."[204] More to the point, it connected cigarettes to images of a lifestyle free of conventional constraints. To some women, that may have been the basis of cigarettes' appeal.

Montez and Carmen were avatars of an idea: women were not just embodiments of cookie-cutter roles: they had personalities, individualities, and rights.[205] The same year that *Carmen* debuted, an ad in *Harper's* by Vanity Fair cigarettes spoke directly to women (or, at least, some women) offering monogrammed cigarettes in

---

[202] *Harper's* published a fascinating survey of women shown to be smoking. See Coffin Nails: The tobacco controversy in the 19th century, https://tobacco.harpweek.com/hubpages/CommentaryPage.asp?Commentary=Women

[203] Amos A & Haglund M. (2010) From social taboo to 'torch of freedom': The marketing of cigarettes to women. *Tob Contr* **9**(38), 3.

[204] Coffin Nails, supra

[205] Starting in the mid-19th century, women were organizing for equal rights. See, e.g., https://history.house.gov/Exhibitions-and-Publications/WIC/Historical-Essays/No-Lady/Womens-Rights/; Brown J.K. (1993) The Nineteenth Amendment and women's equality. *Yale L J* **102**(8), 2175–2204.

small sizes "expressly for ladies."[206] Though women could still be stigmatized for smoking — smoking was louche, unwomanly, a sign of sexual impurity — the ad calibrates any whiff of transgression to women's ostensible delicacy, implying that women could have it both ways.

Women *were* smoking, if still just in limited numbers. In 1885, the Women's Christian Temperance Union identified "ladies' smoking clubs" in several cities.[207] In the 1890s, at least one hotel in New York City had a women's smoking room "to accommodate the practice among its upper-crust patrons."[208] The type of society woman in a Henry James novel could have returned from a European caprice — smoking. She would have become another New Woman, flaunting her independence, challenging traditional gender roles.[209] This "new-ness" had consequences. By the early 20th century, trains had smoking cars for women; amidst the still-vocal disapproval of women's smoking, women had asked for them (probably to escape the male gaze and to socialize with like-minded peers). As Allan Brandt observes, "Antitobacco rhetoric directed at women inevitably created certain appeals for smoking. No doubt, many American women began to experiment with cigarettes long before the glare of advertising would be turned directly up on them." As early as 1916, observers noted a significant rise in

---

[206] Harper's survey, https://tobacco.harpweek.com/hubpages/CommentaryPage.asp?Commentary=Women

[207] https://tobacco.harpweek.com/hubpages/CommentaryPage.asp?Commentary=Women

[208] Id.

[209] See Elliot R. (2005) *Women and Smoking Since 1890*. Routledge, observing that when some intellectual and society women took up smoking in the 1890s, they enacted the emancipation of the "New Woman."

consumption among women."[210] The federal government reported that in FY1917, tobacco sales had increased 15%, due largely to more women smoking.

Cigarette smoking was breaking down how women thought about gender roles. As Brandt observes:

> By the early 20th century, the cigarette had come to represent a powerful clash of cultural values. Traditional morality configured the cigarette as a threat to the moral sanctity of women; at the same time, the cigarette marked the erosion of certain expectations of strict boundaries between the worlds of men and women. The cigarette became a symbol of new roles and expectations of women's behavior.[211]

While men may have seamlessly transitioned from smoking cigarettes in the trenches to smoking them at home, the trajectory was different for women. It represented a transformation, not just in *how* they satisfied the yearn for nicotine but in how — or, rather, whether — they satisfied traditional expectations concerning their deportment. This is why the history of women's turn toward smoking cigarettes cannot just be mapped onto that of men. It was a major cultural upheaval that didn't just happen, full-blown, after the war's end. Rather, favorable conditions had been developing since the mid- to late 19th century and intensified into the 20th century.

After World War I, cigarettes were marketed unabashedly to women. Lucky Strike, for instance, told women "To keep a slender figure No one can deny… reach for a Lucky instead of a sweet."

---

[210] Brandt A. (1996) Recruiting women smokers: The engineering of consent. *J Am Med Womens Assoc* **51**(1–2), 63–66, 63.

[211] Id., 64.

Another ad featured Grace, Lady Hay Drummond-Hay, declaring, "I smoke a Lucky instead of eating sweets." These appeals channeled the flapper obsession with skinniness. See Anne Ewbank's article, "Looking like a flapper meant a diet of celery and cigarettes."[212] Ewbank observes that "smoking distinguished flappers from their mothers and grandmothers, and cigarettes' appetite-suppressing qualities were considered an asset… Marketing cigarettes as slimming agents for young women remained standard for years."[213] It was, moreover, highly successful, and increased Lucky's share of the market by over 200%.[214]

The actress Betty Compson (*The Docks of New York*, *The White Shadow*, *Street Girl*) endorsed Luckies, showcasing the connection between smoking and Hollywood figures of the era. Of course, the most glamorous actress of them all, Marlene Dietrich, smoked through her movies. During the 1920s and 30s, Hollywood frequently portrayed smoking as glamorous and sophisticated.[215] Tobacco companies collaborated with film studios, paying actors to smoke in movies.

---

[212] Ewbanks (2018), in *Gastro Obscura*, https://www.atlasobscura.com/articles/1920s-food-flapper-diet, noting that "the flapper look was lean and androgynous, and maintaining that ideal often required a special 'flapper' diet."

[213] For an extensive discussion of cigarette marketing directed at women, see Christensen W. (2012) Torches of freedom: Women and smoking propaganda, https://thesocietypages.org/socimages/2012/02/27/torches-of-freedom-women-and-smoking-propaganda/. See also Jenson PM. (1994) A history of women and smoking, *Canadian Woman Studies/les cahiers de la femme*.

[214] Amos and Haglund, supra, 4.

[215] On tobacco companies' involvement with Hollywood, see Timeline of tobacco industry Hollywood involvement, https://smokefreemedia.ucsf.edu/history/timeline

But suppose you weren't impressed by those hard-sell ads. There was a cigarette ad for you too. Chesterfield showed a fur-draped, refined young woman confessing, "I really don't know if I should smoke," (what candor!) who then allays her concerns (again with faux candor):

> . . . but my brothers and my sweet-heart smoke, and it does giveme a lot of pleasure.
>
> Women began to smoke, so they tell me, just about the time they began to vote, but that's hardly a reason for women smoking. I guess I just like to smoke, that's all.
>
> It so happens that I smoke CHESTERFIELD. They seem to be milder and they have a very pleasing taste.

The ad targets non-flappers, women who may be somewhat older. The speaker is not a New Woman. She doesn't connect smoking with her rights (as when women "began to vote"). Instead, she looks to two males ("my brothers and my sweet-heart"); decides that, like them, she likes smoking; and then endorses Chesterfield because they "seem" milder (it's so reassuringly casual that you think she's been quoted spontaneously). But wait! She's an artful invention! This very clever ad suggests that women can exercise prerogatives circumspectly, without flouting convention. Choosing to smoke can be a *safe* choice — as safe as just caring for yourself. The reader is made so comfortable that she may give Chesterfield a try. Of course, the ad demonstrates the sophistication of cigarette advertising. If more women had taken up smoking, it may have been on account of such ads.

Section

2 Neuroscience — Drugs of Abuse

The previous section examined the origins of four salient addictive drugs. This section examines the chemical make-up of an array of such drugs, as well as the neuroscience behind them, i.e., the brain mechanisms that determine their effects.

Most people using these drugs do not know what they look like chemically, and how they work in the brain. So, this section introduces this type of scientific material, although we have sought to avoid unnecessary scientific terms and dense scientific referencing. The figures add clarity.

We first begin with opioids, where, as Damaris Albores-Garcia and Silvia L. Cruz explain, the opioid crisis occurred in waves over the last 30 years: "First it began in the late 1990s and was caused by opioid over-prescription, mainly of extended-release oxycodone (OxyContin). The second wave began around 2010 when a significant proportion of patients with chronic pain who had developed opioid use disorder (OUD) switched to heroin. Third, the increased presence of heroin laced with fentanyl and fentanyl analogs triggered a new and deadly wave of the opioid crisis in 2013."[1] We begin by discussing morphine, a natural opium derivative, and then move on to the more dangerous, synthetic opioids cited by Albores-Garcia and Cruz. These will

[1] Albores-García D & Cruz SL. (2023) Fentanyl and other new psychoactive synthetic opioids. Challenges to prevention and treatment. *Revista de investigación clínica* **75**(3), 93–104.

include heroin, a semi-synthetic opioid. We will then examine several other, non-opioid synthetics, e.g., lysergic acid diethylamide (LSD), ketamine, and methamphetamine.

In each case, we illustrate how these drugs work in the brain and why they can become addictive. Our objective, of course, is to help you understand the real, physiological threats posed by these drugs. Additionally, you will be better able to understand current approaches to treating addiction and (in the following section) prospects for finally overcoming addiction.

I. Natural Opium Derivative: Morphine

Morphine is a natural opioid, i.e., a component of opium, and is therefore distinct from other opioids that are synthesized in a lab. Morphine is a potent analgesic, i.e., it is used medically as a painkiller, even though it can be addictive. By comparison, the opioid compound heroin is a street drug and, while it also has analgesic properties, it is not used in clinical settings because it is *highly* addictive.

A juice can be extracted from the poppy plant (Papaver somniferum, opium) that contains morphine (which, in turn, can be used to produce heroin). Besides relieving pain, morphine and heroin may, at some doses, also produce a euphoric state. Additionally, morphine can lower blood pressure, the rate of breathing, and the heart rate. According to the Drug Enforcement Agency (DEA), overdoses of morphine or heroin can be lethal.[2] So, how do opioid chemicals work to achieve their behavioral effects? What is going on in the brain such that they reduce pain and more? They work by engaging proteins in the brain called *opioid receptors*.

---

[2] Drug Enforcement Agency, https://www.dea.gov/factsheets/heroin

Morphine, mu opioid receptor

Morphine is a complex compound with five rings and a molecular weight of 285. Its physiological and behavioral effects derive from its ability to bind to a class of proteins in nerve cell membranes. These proteins are long strings of amino acids that wind back and forth across nerve cell membranes seven times. The concept is that they form an "opioid binding cavity." The three classical types of opioid receptors utilize different parts of the cavity, and different amino acids in the proteins, to render the effects of activating a (1) mu receptor, (2) kappa receptor, or (3) delta opioid receptor (all discussed below).

According to a hypothesis of Maria Waldhoer and her colleagues at the Gallo Center of the University of California, San Francisco, specific divergences in the extracellular loops of these proteins can help to determine selectivity of the receptor for a mu receptor ligand (a substance that binds to a receptor), as compared to a kappa or delta ligand.[3] Then a small ligand such as morphine, meaning a compound with relatively few atoms, which will bind (ligand) to an opioid receptor, would interact mainly with amino acids at the bottom of the opioid binding cavity. In contrast, large delta opioid ligands fill almost all the available space within the opioid receptor.

A classic mu opioid receptor ligand is morphine. Endogenous ligands — chemical compounds produced naturally in the brain — for the different receptor types are: beta-endorphins (mu opioid receptor), enkephalins (delta opioid receptor), and dynorphins (kappa opioid receptor).

---

[3]Waldhoer M, Bartlett SE, & Whistler JL. (2004) Opioid receptors. *Ann Rev Biochem* **73**(1), 953–990.

Activation of the mu opioid receptor leads to analgesia (pain reduction) and sedation. Electrophysiologist Graeme Henderson, at the University of Bristol, has documented neuronal membrane hyperpolarization through opening of potassium channels in the nerve cell membrane — this effect would tend to silence neurons.[4] Such inhibitory effects of mu receptor activation are widespread in the nervous system, but some neurons behave otherwise. As a side point, it has recently been claimed that fentanyl-induced respiratory depression may be mediated by peripheral mu opioid receptors, that is, receptors in the body but outside the brain.

Kappa opioid receptors: ligand example = dynorphin

Activation of kappa receptors reduces pain, but can also lead to dysphoria, hallucinations, and addiction. Different opioids binding to different opioid receptors have different mental and behavioral effects.

The review by Takemori and Portoghese states that specific amino acids in the second extracellular loop of the receptor, negatively charged (that is, containing atoms with excess electrons), are important for efficient kappa ligand binding.[5]

Johns Hopkins scientists Doss and Barrett have studied salvinorinA, the most potent, selective, and effective kappa opioid receptor (KOR) ligand known. They measured connectivity in the

---

[4] Gill H, Kelly E, & Henderson G. (2019) How the complex pharmacology of the fentanyls contributes to their lethality. *Addiction (Abingdon, England)* **114**(9), 1524.

[5] Takemori AE & Portoghese PS. (1992) Selective naltrexone-derived opioid receptor antagonists. *Ann Rev Pharmacol Toxicol* **32**, 239–269.

human brain using functional magnetic resonance imaging (fMRI) minutes after salvinorinA administration (compared to placebo control). In their view, the most prominent effect (of the kappa receptor agonist, the compound activating the KOR) was the attenuation of the default mode network (DMN), referring to a brain network discovered by Marcus Raichle (Washington University, Saint Louis) that is active when the subject is not focused on a specific task but is quietly awake. This is important because the DMN is a fundamental network underlying one aspect of forebrain activity.

Side point: Some molecular pharmacologists envision KOR antagonists as novel therapeutics for major depressive disorders and other stress-related disorders.

Delta receptors: ligand example = enkephalin

Activation of delta receptors also reduces pain. In addition, there is the possibility that delta receptor ligands could have useful antidepressant properties. Note once again that different opioid chemical compounds working at different types of opioid receptors have different mental and behavioral effects.

Delta receptor ligands are thought to engage most of the opioid binding cavity (see above). More definitive results are awaited. In addition, they are thought to interact with specific amino acids — valine, arginine, and tryptophan in the third extracellular loop of the receptor protein — as well as the amino acid asparagine in the second transmembrane segment. Delta receptor binding may have important properties as an antidepressant.

Antidepressant effects of an opioid receptor ligand can be inhibited in the presence of the delta-selective "antagonist" (it blocks delta receptor function — the opposite of "agonist"), confirming the involvement of the delta receptor in protecting against depression.

Heroin

Heroin is derived from morphine by adding two small chemical groups. It has a molecular weight of 369 and is an unremarkable-looking ringed organic compound. It is much more lipophilic (it dissolves easily in lipids, i.e., fat) than morphine and passes the blood–brain barrier much faster. When metabolized to monoacetylmorphine and back to morphine, it works powerfully through the mu opioid receptor within nerve cells in the brain and nerve cells in the spinal cord. Through these actions, it reduces pain. It can also be used to produce euphoria. Overdoses, as mentioned above, can be fatal.

As with virtually all addictive drugs, morphine and heroin can produce serious withdrawal symptoms in those seeking to quit. The initial painful withdrawal syndrome peaks within a few days and can persist for several months. The primary strategy for dealing with the painful symptoms (anxiety, sweating, vomiting, muscle aches) is the chronic administration of long-acting opioids, methadone and buprenorphine. Of course, the next step is to prevent resumption of use with naltrexone, a long-acting mu opioid receptor antagonist. Psychotherapeutic interventions such as cognitive behavioral therapy are also useful.

Overall, the actions of opioids are a complex topic involving an array of substances with helpful and harmful attributes, where the former can tip into the latter when the drugs are used indiscriminately. The subject is also complex, regarding the molecular pharmacology of opioid peptide actions.

II. Fentanyl

Fentanyl is a synthetic opioid that is made in a lab from precursor chemicals. There are two sources of fentanyl: (1) pharmaceutical fentanyl, which is produced legally and is prescribed by doctors to manage severe pain, e.g., after surgery, and (2) illicitly manufactured fentanyl, produced in secretive labs and distributed by illegal drug dealers. In the latter case, consumers may be unaware that they are taking fentanyl, since it is often mixed with (and sold as) other drugs, which is most insidious, because tiny amounts of fentanyl can be toxic and the results can be disastrous when such amounts are illicitly mixed into other drugs. Fentanyl can be smuggled into the country in innocent-looking containers.

The problem. The National Institute on Drug Abuse states that deaths in the United States (U.S.) related to synthetic opioids (mainly fentanyl) rose to over 70,000 in 2021, whereas in 2019 they had been ~40,000. That's an increase of 75% in 2 years! The Centers for Disease Control and Prevention (CDC) reported 75,000 synthetic opioid deaths in 2022, again with fentanyl the main culprit.

Fentanyl is a common adulterant in street drugs, such as heroin, prescription pain pills, and sedatives. Fentanyl-adulterated cocaine and methamphetamine also contribute to rising numbers of deaths.

Fentanyl can be used as an anesthetic and to reduce pain. But here, we focus on it as a drug of abuse because, on the street, it is illicit — it began as a substitute for heroin. While it can produce euphoria, it can kill by depressing respiration.

Because fentanyl is so potent, it is easy to smuggle, i.e., it is easy to hide because small amounts of the drug produce strong effects. Thus, traffickers have increasingly turned to fentanyl because it is cheap to produce; it can be marked up many times the original cost. Moreover, the chemistry of fentanyl is not complicated; it can be manufactured illicitly by under-the-radar operations, not only in the U.S. but also, for example, in Mexico and China. More than 20 fentanyl derivatives are manufactured, making it even harder to suppress or even keep track of.

In addition, it is slow to be eliminated from the body. Multiple doses of the opioid blocker naloxone (see below) are sometimes required before a consumer is safely clear of it.

On May 25, 2023, the House of Representatives passed legislation that would permanently list fentanyl-related drugs (several drugs chemically similar to fentanyl) as Schedule I controlled substances, a designation that mandates severe prison sentences for selling or distributing highly addictive, nonmedicinal chemicals. This designation expired at the end of 2024, and it is now a Schedule II drug — still with a high potential for abuse. The issue of its designation is fraught, however, because some in Congress argue that increased penalties will only push up drug-related incarceration rates that mainly affect people of color.

Some technical details. Of the three opioid receptors in the brain, fentanyl and its derivatives bind to the mu opioid receptors that mediate respiratory depression. Fentanyl is 50 to 100 times more potent than morphine or heroin. This may be due partly to the fact that it interacts with the mu opioid receptors, not only by a commonly found type of "ionic bond" (with transfer of electrons) but also through an additional connection, a stable "hydrogen bond."

Importantly, fentanyl is "lipophilic". Since our brains are full of lipids, and since fentanyl crosses the blood–brain-barrier, it can deliver a whoppingly fast knockout punch to parts of our brain responsible for managing respiration and, indeed, levels of consciousness.

Fentanyl withdrawal symptoms (sweating, restlessness, joint aches, gastrointestinal upset, tremor, anxiety, irritability) are managed with approaches like those for opioid withdrawal. But fentanyl withdrawal may be more uncomfortable and difficult, leading to increased challenges around engagement in recovery programs and retention (e.g., staying in the programs) for those experiencing it. Methadone (see below) is usually part of a comprehensive regimen of withdrawal treatment, but it is not uncommon that long-acting buprenorphine (also see below) is necessary to manage withdrawal symptoms.

Some questions. Clearly, education regarding this drug is crucial. The more that people know about it, the more they will be on guard. Are children adequately educated about opioids? Can medical care in prisons be improved so that prisoners do not develop a drug habit while incarcerated, in an effort to self-medicate? Can opioid receptor blockers like naloxone be made more accessible (some, but not all, states allow access to naloxone without a prescription)? Can we train more social workers in treating opioid addiction?

III. Carfentanil

Of all the fentanyl-related opioids, carfentanil is perhaps the most dangerous. Its chemistry is the same as fentanyl, with a single chemical side chain added. Think of the danger this way. If fentanyl is about 100 times more potent than morphine in terms of depressing respiration and blood pressure and blocking consciousness, then carfentanil is 50 times more potent than fentanyl. Carfentanil is a killer. It was meant for anesthesia in elephants.

Carfentanil is especially dangerous because, as in the case of fentanyl, users may not be aware of its presence. Alan D. Kaye, at Louisiana State University Health Science Center, warns that carfentanil is "commonly found as an additive in other illicit drugs such as heroin and cocaine, meaning many unwitting users may be completely unaware of its presence. As carfentanil is not regularly tested for in most routine drug screening panels, investigators are still unsure of the extent to which it contributes to yearly opioid overdose deaths."[6]

Carfentanil crosses the blood–brain barrier and acts on neurons by binding to proteins called "opioid receptors." As mentioned in the discussion of morphine and heroin, there are three types of opioid receptors: mu, kappa, and delta. By far, cafentanil has the highest affinity for the mu opioid receptor, binding to it roughly 100 times more than the other opioid receptors. Its high affinity for the mu receptor can account for its high toxicity.

It's strange. On the one hand, in terms of brain physiology, fentanyl acts like a super-morphine, though its chemical configuration does not look like morphine's. On the other hand, while carfentanil is much more potent than fentanyl, its chemistry looks almost identical, with just an added oxygen atom in a large (molecular weight is 394) molecule.

How can we explain the lethal power of carfentanil? There are two chemical linkages to consider: (1) its binding to the mu opioid receptor, and (2) the binding of the mu opioid receptor to proteins under the nerve cell membrane. This summary rests on the landmark review by the University of Bristol's Graeme Henderson, Eamonn Kelly, and their team.[7]

Binding. Carfentanil binds with higher affinity than fentanyl to the mu opioid receptor and is much more potent in

---

[6] Edinoff AN, Martinez Garza D, Vining SP, *et al.* (2023) New synthetic opioids: Clinical considerations and dangers. *Pain Thera* **12**(2), 399–421.

[7] Gill H, Kelly E, & Henderson G. (2019) How the complex pharmacology of the fentanyls contributes to their lethality. *Addiction* **14**(9), 1524–1525.

causing physiological effects. It is bound to the receptor within 5 minutes, and then it slowly dissociates from that receptor. As the Kelly-Henderson group at the University of Bristol reported, the effects of carfentanil are more difficult to reverse with naloxone than, e.g., morphine. One peculiarity of this action is that it seems to divest the nerve cell surface of mu opioid receptors for some time, an unusual phenomenon of unknown significance.

Signaling to intracellular proteins. The previous observations are interesting drug-binding facts, but they don't seem striking enough to explain carfentanil's role as a killer. For a better explanation, we look to the mu receptor's relationship to the proteins under the nerve cell membrane. These proteins are called G-proteins because they are guanine (G, as in DNA's G<A<T<C) nucleotide-binding proteins. These proteins can either activate intracellular signaling pathways culminating in gene transcription, or inhibit them. When G-protein signaling has been turned on, it needs to be turned off in some cases. That is the function of another set of membrane-associated proteins called arrestins. It turns out that carfentanil, bound to the mu opioid receptor, signals preferentially through one of these arrestins: beta arrestin 2. Immunoelectron microscopy shows that the beta-arrestins are appropriately situated at postsynaptic sites, in place to regulate G protein-coupled neurotransmitter receptors.

Odds are that this feature of carfentanil's lethality has something to do with this intracellular signaling. But as to how that occurs, i.e., the next steps beyond Beta arrestin 2, we don't yet know.

Regarding withdrawal from carfentanil, Anthony Phillips and Michael Krausz of the University of British Columbia see two patterns. Sometimes, withdrawal proceeds with minimal muscular pain and little vomiting and diarrhea. More often, intervention with an "approved opioid" is necessary. That means the use of methadone or buprenorphine is necessary. These opioids occupy the mu opioid receptor for a lengthy period, thus blocking out the carfentanil.[8]

In summary, as Kara Lynch, at the University of California, San Francisco, observed in 2018, "fentanyl use is increasing due to illicit pills, ease of purchase, and contamination of the North American heroin supply. And as soon as opioids are regulated, new synthetic opioids appear, making detection difficult and the number of cases underreported."[9]

Looking forward, Sylvia Cruz advocates greater surveillance for monitoring drug trends, raising awareness about the risks associated with opioid use through public health alerts, drug checking services, and syringe exchange programs, as well as other harm reduction strategies.

IV. Lysergic Acid Diethylamide (LSD)

Lysergic acid diethylamide (LSD), a complicated-looking multi-ringed compound, is classified as "psychedelic," meaning that it can produce hallucinations and other alterations of consciousness. LSD, which is water soluble, readily crosses the blood–brain barrier (a layering of nerve cells, glial cells, and lipids), and can have psychological effects within minutes, including some that users

---

[8] Phillips AG & Krausz MR. (2018) Utilizing resources of neuropsychopharmacology to address the opioid overdose crisis. *Neuropsychopharmacol Rep* **38**(3), 100–104.

[9] Armenian P, Vo KT, Barr-Walker J, & Lynch KL. (2018) Fentanyl, fentanyl analogs and novel synthetic opioids: A comprehensive review. *Neuropharmacology* **134**, 121–132.

refer to as "mystical" experiences. Some people enjoy the hallucinations; they experience a "good trip." Negative reactions include anxiety and, more seriously, paranoia.

According to the DEA research guide, users may experience changes in their visual worlds as well as extreme changes in mood. Impaired perception (including hallucinations) in several sensory dimensions (vision, hearing, olfaction, etc.) is to be expected. These likely symptoms could produce impaired judgment. The DEA guide also focuses on anxiety and depression after an LSD trip, sometimes days and weeks afterward.

Concerning: Both LSD and psilocybin (see below) share structural similarities with medications that raise the risk of cardiac fibrosis.

A practice called "microdosing" most commonly involves ingesting sub-threshold doses of LSD. Vince Polito and his team evaluated methodological gaps and challenges in microdosing research and suggest several reasons why current claims about microdosing are suspect, including the small number of controlled studies, small sample sizes, susceptibility to selection bias, among other shortcomings.[10]

History. According to David Nichols, at the University of North Carolina, the discovery of LSD as a psychoactive drug occurred accidentally during a period of interest in the neurochemistry of mental disorders.[11] However, progress on understanding LSD was interrupted by the unintended and dangerous use of the drug for recreational purposes.

---

[10] Polito V & Liknaitzky P. (2022) The emerging science of microdosing: A systematic review of research on low dose psychedelics (1955–2021) and recommendations for the field. *Neurosci Biobehav Rev* **139**, 104706.

[11] Nichols DE. (2016) Psychedelics. *Pharmacol Rev* **68**(2), 264–355.

LSD is now being investigated for the treatment of psychiatric disorders, such as depression and anxiety. Clinical trials with psilocybin and LSD have shown improvement in emotional and psychological scores on tests of well-being.[12] Although these drugs are reported to be safe in a controlled environment (such as clinical trials), we are concerned about chronic exposures, such as in workplaces.

Network mechanisms. LSD can alter functional networks in the brain. Yet the detailed mechanisms underpinning the neurobiological response to LSD are still being worked out. The strongest set of data so far has to do with the DMN, a network of forebrain regions, which, as studied with magnetic resonance imaging (MRI), are most active when the subject is at rest with no task assigned. Discovered in the lab of Marcus Raichle at Washington University of Saint Louis, as noted above, the DMN is what Raichle calls "task negative."[13] LSD reduces activity in the DMN; DMN activity is anticorrelated with a forebrain "attention network," activated during attention-demanding tasks. Thus, "task positive."

LSD has led to decreased connectivity within the DMN and increased sensory and thalamocortical connectivity. Correlations between these neurophysiological changes and subjective experiences were noted by clinicians, suggesting a brain network basis of the psychedelics' psychological impacts. For example, according to James Gattuso and his team, there is consistent acute disruption in resting state connectivity within the DMN with LSD:

---

[12] Videira NB, Nair V, Paquet V, & Calhoun D. (2024).The changing outlook of psychedelic drugs: The importance of risk assessment and occupational exposure limits. *J Appl Toxicol* **44**(2), 216–234.

[13] Fox MD, Snyder AZ, Vincent JL, *et al.* (2005) The human brain is intrinsically organized into dynamic, anticorrelated functional networks, *Proc Nat Acad Sci* **102**(27), 9673–9678.

"Altered connectivity in the DMN has been associated with a range of neuropsychiatric conditions such as depression, anxiety, post-traumatic stress disorder, attention deficit/hyperactivity disorder, schizophrenia, and obsessive-compulsive disorder."[14]

George Mashour's lab at the University of Michigan listed eight types of networks, including Default Mode, Attention, and Salience networks, and found that across the board, LSD reduces within-network functional connectivity while enhancing between-network functional connectivity.[15] The ultimate psychological meaning of these results remains to be discovered.

Biochemical mechanisms. Pharmacologically, LSD can cause hallucinations by stimulating cortical serotonin 5-HT_{2A} receptors, although whether 5-HT_{2A} is responsible for the manifestation of any therapeutic effects remains unclear. Daniel Wacker demonstrates that psychedelics like LSD bind to types of nerve cell membrane proteins called "G protein coupled receptors" to initiate signaling, which elicits their physiological actions.[16] While the most frequently discussed mechanism for LSD involves its positive actions through the serotonin 5-HT_{2A} receptor, it also binds to other serotonin receptors and even dopamine receptors D1 and D2.

An additional mechanism of LSD action was discovered in the Helsinki lab of Eero Castren.[17] LSD can act by binding to TrkB, the

---

[14] Gattuso JJ, *et al.* (2023) Default mode network modulation by psychedelics: A systematic review. *Int J Neuropsychopharmacol* **26**(3):155–188.

[15] Lee U & Mashour GA. (2018) Role of network science in the study of anesthetic state transitions. *Anesthesiology* **129**(5), 1029–1044.

[16] Wacker D, Wang S, McCorvy JD, *et al.* (2017) Crystal structure of an LSD-bound human serotonin receptor. *Cell* **168**(3), 377–389.e12.

[17] Moliner R, Girych M, Brunello CA, *et al.* (2023) Psychedelics promote plasticity by directly binding to BDNF receptor TrkB. *Nat Neurosci* **26**(6), 1032–1041.

receptor for the brain-derived neurotrophic factor (BDNF). "The effects of psychedelics on neurotrophic signaling, plasticity, and antidepressant-like behavior in mice depend on TrkB binding and promotion of endogenous BDNF signaling but are independent of serotonin 2A receptor (5-HT_{2A}) activation." So, both 5-HT_{2A} and non-5-HT_{2A} are involved in the behavioral effects of LSD.

Why does all this matter? At least in part, because of the longevity of this drug's popularity. Interest in LSD exploded because of the popularity (and loquacity) of Timothy Leary and other Harvard professors during the 1960s. Although its popularity has rested on its recreational use, the possibility of medical use has not been ruled out. After a long period during which LSD was avoided in science labs, psychedelic-assisted psychotherapy is getting a new look.

As a side point, because the danger of hallucinations limits more widespread therapeutic use of psychedelics as potential antidepressants, new work has focused on a non-hallucinogenic LSD analog: 2-bromo-LSD (2-Br-LSD). 2-Br-LSD binds to 5-HT_{2A} receptors and does not cause some of the unwanted behavioral effects in lab animals.

Methodological considerations. Rachel Yehuda and her coauthors have provided a comprehensive critical assessment of the ability of LSD and other psychedelics to treat post-traumatic stress disorder (PTSD).[18] After a history of the psychiatric use of LSD, these authors warn about potential anxiety, panic, or nausea following LSD. In this difficult type of research, she worries about the complications of patients' expectancies and the absence of

---

[18]Zaretsky TG, Jagodnik KM, Barsic R, *et al.* (2024) The psychedelic future of post-traumatic stress disorder treatment. *Curr Neuropharmacol* **22**(4), 636–735.

sample populations, which are representative of the public's diversity. So far, this research does not come up to the gold standard: the randomized, double-blind crossover clinical trial.

At Brown University, Carolina Haass-Koffler particularly warns of the methodological problem that traditional placebo administration is insufficient to control for expectancy confounds. "Consequently, experimental methodology that limits personnel unblinding and the use of an active placebo are important considerations when designing prospective clinical studies involving psychedelics."[19]

In terms of withdrawal from LSD, about 9% of subjects in one study reported lingering cognitive impairment; almost 3% reported seeking psychiatric or psychological assistance if they had had a "bad trip." Apparently, these problems do not show up with microdosing.

V. Psilocybin

Compared to research on the other drugs discussed here, the literature is quite thin on the mushroom-derivative psilocybin, its brain mechanisms, and its behavior. However, some researchers hope that psilocybin will be useful, and have generated a small wave of enthusiasm about this "psychedelic" drug (so called because it can produce hallucinations and apparent alterations of consciousness). Its apparent attractions are like those of LSD.

Psilocybin (Fig. 1) is a relatively small, simple organic chemical (in technical detail, 3-[2-(Dimethylamino)ethyl]-1H-indol-4-yl

---

[19] Haass-Koffler CL & Schank JR. (2020) Translational research in the neurobiological mechanisms of alcohol and substance use disorders. *Neurotherapeutics* **17**(1), 1–3.

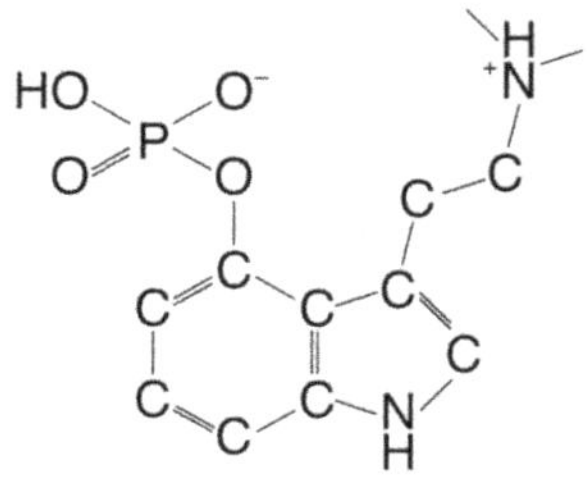

Fig. 1. Psilocybin. This "psychedelic" drug, distributed widely in the brain, causes disorientation.

dihydrogen phosphate) featuring two carbonaceous rings and a phosphate group in a chemical structure similar to serotonin's. Different strengths of psilocybin can be derived from various mushrooms. It is water-soluble. Its active metabolite (with the phosphate group removed) is psilocin.

Psilocybin readily crosses the blood–brain barrier and is widely distributed in the brain. The team led by Paul Hutson at the University of Wisconsin showed that oral administration is followed by peak concentrations in the blood 2–3 hours later, sinking to very low levels by 12 hours.[20] Yale researchers Davoudian and Kwan reported psilocybin-induced expression of the c-Fos gene, usually correlated with increased electrical activity, in widespread areas of the lab animal brain: anterior cingulate cortex, locus coeruleus, primary visual cortex, central and basolateral amygdala, medial and lateral habenula, and claustrum.[21]

---

[20] Brown RT, Nicholas CR, Cozzi NV, *et al.* (2017). Pharmacokinetics of escalating doses of oral psilocybin in healthy adults. *Clin Pharmacokinet* **56**(12), 1543–1554.

[21] Davoudian PA, Shao LX, & Kwan AC. (2023) Shared and distinct brain regions targeted for immediate early gene expression by ketamine and psilocybin. *ACS Chem Neurosci* **14**(3), 468–480.

Behavioral effects in human subjects are highly variable and depend on the social environment and physical atmosphere, but they always include disorientation and emotional swings. Psychological effects are at a maximum at about 2 hours and last 5–6 hours. David Olson's group at the University of California, Davis, highlighted drug effects on circuits relevant to mood, fear, reward, and cognitive flexibility.[22]

Mechanisms

Psilocybin's effects on the brain are intimately related to serotonin, which means that we face a complex situation: No fewer than 14 receptors for serotonin have been identified in nerve cells. These are grouped into seven families and include some that are excitatory and others that are inhibitory. Further, activation of serotonin receptors can modulate the release of other neurotransmitters. Complex indeed.

Psilocybin's actions have been convincingly tied to the serotonin receptor called 5HT2A. Deepak Cyril D'Souza's lab at Yale reported that psilocin, the active metabolite, binds to 5HT2A about five times more than any other serotonin receptor tested. Antagonism of the 5HT2A receptor blocks the psychedelic effects.[23] 5HT2A has targets widespread throughout the body and is connected to a variety of physiological and behavioral functions. Its physiology is complicated. First, the receptor can have constitutive activity, e.g., on learning, in the absence of a serotonergic agonist. Second, it is

---

[22] Saeger HN & Olson DE. (2022) Psychedelic-inspired approaches for treating neurodegenerative disorders. *J Neurochem* **162**(1): 109–127.

[23] Holze F, Singh N, Liechti ME, & D'Souza DC. (2024) Serotonergic psychedelics: A comparative review of efficacy, safety, pharmacokinetics, and binding profile. *Biol Psychiatry Cogn Neurosci Neuroimaging* **9**(5), 472–489.

involved in aspects of neurophysiology as varied as those connected to depression, schizophrenia, suicide, reward, and movement.

Useful?

Investigations into the possible medical usefulness of psilocybin have generated hope that it could combat depression and reduce pain. Regarding depression, Roland Griffiths' lab at Johns Hopkins has run the gold standard of clinical trials: randomized controlled trials in which the patient does not know whether (s)he has received the psychedelic drug.[24] Compared to controls, patients receiving psilocybin reported, through a standardized depression questionnaire, a highly statistically significant reduction in symptoms of depression.

Charles Raison, at Wisconsin, led a large collaborative team in a randomized, placebo-controlled trial where psilocybin, administered with psychological support, was associated with a rapid and sustained antidepressant effect. No serious treatment-emergent adverse events occurred. Reviews by Tessa Watford and Naqash Masood at Keele University in the United Kingdom (U.K.) and Istanbul University's Nur Damla Korkmaz support the conclusion that there is a role for psilocybin in combating depression.[25]

Pain. The types of chronic pain addressed successfully by psilocybin have been lower back pain, cluster headache disorders,

---

[24] Raison CL, Sanacora G, Woolley J, *et al.* (2023) Single-dose psilocybin treatment for major depressive disorder: A randomized clinical trial. *JAMA* **330**(9), 843–853.

[25] Watford T & Masood N. (2024) Psilocybin, an effective treatment for major depressive disorder in adults — a systematic review. *Clin Psychopharmacol Neurosci* **22**(1), 2–12; Korkmaz ND, *et al.* (2024) Psychedelic therapy in depression and substance use disorders. *Eur J Neurosci* **60**(2), 4063–4077.

fibromyalgia, and neuropathic pain. Activation of 5-HT2A via injection of serotonin (5-HT) into the spinal cord results in anti-nociceptive effects, interfering with pain signaling.

An AI-powered review by Christopher L. Robinson, at Harvard Medical School, and University of Pittsburgh's Trent Emerick concluded that "psychedelics such as psilocybin may have potential in alleviating pain symptoms secondary to a multitude of chronic pain conditions."[26] The effects of 5-HT activation are dependent on the specific characteristics of the pain, such as whether it is acute or chronic, and the location of pain activation, whether peripheral or central.

Clearly, the psychological effects of psilocybin are not as comprehensively demonstrated as those of some other chemicals in our discussion. Regulatory reviews at the FDA and elsewhere may be tough to satisfy because of an unfavorable relation of risk to benefit. In view of the significant side effects, which can include nausea, vomiting, and psychotic symptoms, is psilocybin worth it? The jury is still out.

VI. Ketamine

Rather suddenly, ketamine, which is useful medically as an anesthetic, has gained popularity (and notoriety) as a recreational drug. It's time to think about it.

For medical use, ketamine (Fig. 2) is a dissociative anesthetic that can be used, for example, in the treatment of acute pain. (It is "dissociative" because it can distort perception of sight and sound,

---

[26] Robinson CL, Fonseca ACG, Diejomaoh EM, *et al.* (2024) Scoping review: The role of psychedelics in the management of chronic pain. *J Pain Res* **17**, 965–973.

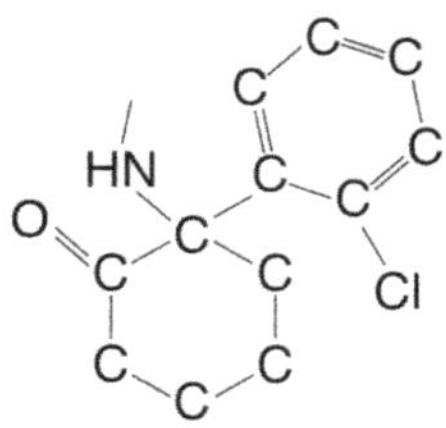

Fig. 2. Ketamine. An anesthetic, ketamine is also a party drug.

and produce feelings of detachment, i.e., dissociation, from the environment and the self). Ketamine can also be used as a rapidly acting antidepressant, especially where other antidepressants have been ineffective.

Ketamine has become a party drug precisely because of its dissociative qualities, allowing users to feel detached from reality, e.g., as in emotional detachment — "I don't care about him." It can also cause hallucinations, perceptual distortions, and, at high doses, unconsciousness. Some have had terrifying "bad trips," similar to delirium. It is potentially harmful and subject to abuse. A few studies indicate that ketamine has the potential to be addictive. A report by the Independent Scientific Committee on Drugs (now known as Drug Science) states that users will keep on using until the supply runs out. Then they may crave the drug and show withdrawal symptoms such as anxiety, shaking, sweating, and palpitations. This is a sign of addiction. Further, there is the "tolerance" phenomenon, where the need for increasing dosage is one index of a substance's addictive potential. By that criterion, ketamine can be addictive.

The synthesis of ketamine is chemically straightforward. That is troubling because Chinese chemists and Mexican cartels can supply the drug cheaply and in large amounts.

How does ketamine work? It is lipid-soluble, so it gets into the brain rapidly and diffuses freely. What kinds of neurons does ketamine address? Mainly, we should think about neurons affected by the excitatory neurotransmitter glutamate and one of its receptor types, the so-called NMDA (N-methyl-D-aspartate) receptor. Picture NMDA receptor subtypes as four proteins in the nerve cell membrane with a pore between them. As reviewed by Todd Gould at the University of Maryland Medical School, ketamine blocks the pore and thus reduces a major excitatory drive on those neurons.[27]

There is also a new mechanism of ketamine's action against depression, thus adding to the NMDA receptor story. There is an enzyme expressed in the brain called "extracellular signal-regulated kinase" (ERK). A kinase is an enzyme that carries out a crucial type of step: adding phosphate groups to other proteins. Ketamine's actions in the brain could be augmented by increasing ERK activity, and that ketamine achieves that result by inhibiting a competing enzyme that takes off those phosphate groups. An important feature of this augmentation is to extend its action in time, thus avoiding unwanted side effects of high-frequency repeated treatments.

Ketamine affects other neurotransmitter receptors as well, including all three types of opioid receptors. It is less clear how those actions contribute to mental and behavioral changes.

Where in the brain does ketamine act against depression? It is understood that depressive conditions do not occur because of

---

[27]Zanos P & Gould TD. (2018) Mechanisms of ketamine action as an antidepressant. *Mol Psychiatry* **23**(4), 801–811.

just one type of biochemical change in just one group of neurons. That said, the cingulate cortex has come in for a lot of attention.

The cingulate cortex comprises neurons along the midline, some of which are folded down in the gap between the left and right hemispheres of the brain. Attention to this area of cortex with respect to depression is due largely to the groundbreaking work of Dr. Helen Mayberg, formerly at Emory and now at Mount Sinai School of Medicine. Mayberg used a combination of techniques, including positron emission tomography (PET scan) and electrical stimulation of the brain, to arrive at the idea that achieving decreased blood flow and reduced metabolic rate in the anterior cingulate cortex, and increased blood flow and metabolic rate in the posterior cingulate cortex, might be ideal for beating treatment-resistant depression. In fact, ketamine reduces CC activation within minutes.[28] This physiological change in ACC correlates with ketamine's antidepressant effects, according to Laith Alexander and his colleagues at King's College London.[29]

Ketamine is complicated — it is useful to physicians but dangerous at parties. The United Nations World Drug Report describes the drug's rapid spread worldwide. So, as with all potentially addictive drugs — even those that can just cause harm when improperly used — people should be educated about the dangers. We also need to combat illicit supply. To the extent that we develop rapid treatments for an overdose (like naloxone for opioids), these should be made readily available.

---

[28] Moreines, JL, McClintock SM, Kelley ME, *et al.* (2014) Neuropsychological function before and after subcallosal cingulate deep brain stimulation in patients with treatment-resistant depression. *Depress Anxiety* **31**(8), 690–698.

[29] Alexander L, Hawkins PCT, Evans JW, *et al.* (2023) Preliminary evidence that ketamine alters anterior cingulate resting-state functional connectivity in depressed individuals. *Transl Psychiatry* **13**(1), 371.

VII. Cocaine

Cocaine addiction is among the earliest, but still one of the most prevalent manifestations of drug abuse in the U.S. While the drug heightens arousal and produces intense feelings of reward, it also negatively affects the autonomic nervous system, e.g., by raising the heart rate and blood pressure.

Neuroscience data on cocaine's biochemical effects in the brain explain why cocaine users become hyper-aroused. By blocking uptake of certain neurotransmitters into nerve cells, cocaine increases extracellular levels of the arousal-elevating neurotransmitters dopamine and norepinephrine.

The dopaminergic input to the reward-associated basal forebrain nucleus accumbens from the midbrain's ventral tegmental area is essential for cocaine-seeking. So-called "medium spiny neurons" in the nucleus accumbens (Fig. 3) feature dopamine receptors, "D1 receptors." These are composed of proteins, which have their components on the outer side of the neuronal cell membrane, as well as within the membrane itself, and finally on the inner side of the membrane. Dopamine binds to the part within the cell membrane, specifically with hydrogen bonds to the amino acids, serine and phenylalanine. This binding is behaviorally important: Mice lacking the gene for the D1 receptor show

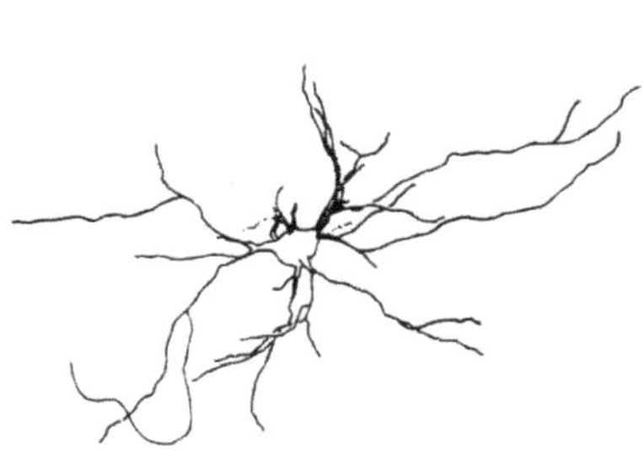

Fig. 3. Spiny neuron. In the basal forebrain's nucleus accumbens, this type of neuron plays a central role in behavioral reward.

no effect of cocaine on arousal. Data from laboratories like Roy Wise's at the National Institute for Drug Abuse (NIDA) show that dopamine effects in the nucleus accumbens play "a crucial role in cocaine self-administration."[30]

On the inner side of the nucleus accumbens nerve cell membrane, the D1 receptor contacts a type of membrane-associated protein called a "G protein," which acts as a molecular switch to turn on a signaling system in the cytoplasm and nucleus of the neurons, which uses a simple biochemical called "cyclic AMP."

What exactly is cocaine doing in the nucleus accumbens and elsewhere in the brain to produce intense addiction? We agree with Pittsburgh neuroscientist Yan Dong that there is no simple, widely accepted summary of the cocaine-induced changes that directly contribute to the addictive state.[31] One possibility is that neurons in the nucleus accumbens and/or VTA dopamine neurons become highly sensitized to the excitatory neurotransmitter glutamate, with the effect of producing a feeling of intense need for the drug.

Another possibility, suggested by Barry Everitt and Trevor Robbins at the University of Cambridge, involves activation of a specific set of motor control neurons in the forebrain beneath the cortex, coupled with decreased executive control over drug-seeking neurons by cells in the prefrontal cortex (PFC) and orbitofrontal cortex.[32] In fact, Nora Volkow, Director of the National Institute on Drug Abuse, and her team reported that cocaine intake markedly

---

[30] Wise RA & Robble MA. (2020) Dopamine and Addiction. *Ann Rev Psychol* **71**, 79–106.

[31] Ahmed SH, Lin D, Koob GF, & Parsons LH. (2003) Escalation of cocaine self-administration does not depend on altered cocaine-induced nucleus accumbens dopamine levels. *J Neurochem* **86**(1), 102–113.

[32] Everitt BJ & Robbins TW. (2016) Drug addiction: Updating actions to habits to compulsions ten years on. *Ann Rev Psychol* **67**, 23–50.

reduced blood flow in the PFC, coupled with attenuated reactivity of neurons located there to electrical stimulation in the midbrain.[33] Others have also shown that cocaine self-administration decreased intrinsic excitability of PFC neurons and, indeed, that PFC stimulation prevented compulsive cocaine seeking.

George Koob, now at NIH's National Institute of Alcohol Abuse and Alcoholism, and Kent Berridge, at the University of Michigan, added a perspective. They suggest that stress is one factor in users' resorting to an addictive chemical like cocaine.[34] Thus, Berridge addresses the neurons that produce the neuropeptide, abbreviated CRF, which regulates an entire hierarchy of stress-reactive hormones. He found that electrically activating CRF-producing neurons in a basal forebrain neuronal group essential for behavioral reward — and other CRF neurons — increased the animal's motivation to pursue cocaine. Berridge noted that other neurotransmitters released from CRF neurons upon stimulation may contribute to the behavioral effect of heightened cocaine seeking. It is important to note that Berridge developed his knowledge of addictive drugs into a coherent theory of drug addiction (see below).

Thus, in cocaine, we have a well-explained phenomenon, cocaine-induced arousal, combined with a more complicated problem — cocaine addiction.

Withdrawal from cocaine: At first, soon after final drug taking, addicts will experience exhaustion, hypersomnia, cravings, and irritability. Other unfortunate consequences of withdrawal are

---

[33] Du C, Volkow ND, You J, *et al.* (2020) Cocaine-induced ischemia in prefrontal cortex is associated with escalation of cocaine intake in rodents. *Mol Psychiatry* **25**(8), 1759–1776.

[34] Koob GF, Buck CL, Cohen A, *et al.* (2014) Addiction as a stress surfeit disorder. *Neuropharmacology* **76**, 370–382.

depression and the inability to enjoy things in life. Later, weeks after stopping use, former addicts will suffer from cognitive dysfunction (e.g., inability to make decisions), lethargy, anxiety, and depression.

VIII. Amphetamine and Methamphetamine

These two stimulants may be sources of pleasure — from euphoria to sex — but can also cause a lot of trouble, i.e., a dependence that may require psychotherapy.

Amphetamine and methamphetamine can cross the blood–brain barrier and, in drug abuse, can degrade the function of the blood–brain barrier: the barrier is broken down, resulting in uncontrolled permeability. Bryan Yamamoto, of the Indiana University School of Medicine, has documented that "compromised blood–brain barrier allows for the unregulated passage of water, proteins, or inflammatory mediators such as macrophages and neutrophils that induce brain edema and can contribute to brain damage or neurodegeneration."[35]

Of course, as a "stimulant," amphetamine increases what elsewhere I have called "generalized CNS [central nervous system] arousal." That is, it increases the amount and speed of movement and sharpens certain cognitive functions such as attention and alertness. According to the DEA, amphetamine use "increases blood pressure and pulse rates, causes insomnia and loss of appetite, and, eventually, physical exhaustion." Amphetamine increases

---

[35] Rodriguez EA & Yamamoto BK. (2021) Toxic effects of methamphetamine on perivascular health: Co-morbid effects of stress and alcohol use disorders. *Curr Neuropharmacol* **19**(12), 2092–2107.

cerebral blood flow, reduces fatigue (until the person is totally exhausted), and reduces appetite.

Amphetamine abuse is associated with a range of neurologic and psychiatric disorders, sometimes accompanied by nerve cell death. One mechanism for this is damage to a subcellular organelle called the endoplasmic reticulum, resulting in improperly folded proteins produced in the nerve cell.

Methamphetamine ("meth") abuse is worse. While the drug has pharmacological actions like those of amphetamine, its potency is greater in the brain than outside it. Bryan Yamamoto notes that the small size and lipophilicity of methamphetamine allow it to spread widely in the brain. The Princeton Detox & Recovery Center states that meth is "highly addictive" and can lead to sudden episodes of euphoria. However, it notes that "because the high doesn't last long, those that experiment with the drug will usually take more within a short time period to prolong the high. When the drug wears off, the user will experience a physical and psychological crash. In order to prevent this crash, the user might take even more meth. Because the vicious cycle happens so quickly, those that experiment with the habit-forming drug — even once — are prone to develop a serious addiction."

The NIDA warns that long-term meth abuse can have serious consequences — paranoia, schizophrenia, anxiety, and depression. But meth is still everywhere. It has become a dangerous street drug. Illegal traffic in meth is the basis of the long-running TV series, *Breaking Bad*, which dramatizes the difficulty of eradicating its production.

Of great clinical interest, on the other hand, Syracuse professor Stephen Faraone highlighted the use of amphetamine as therapy for attention-deficit/hyperactivity disorder (ADHD). In Faraone's words, "The primary pharmacologic effect of both

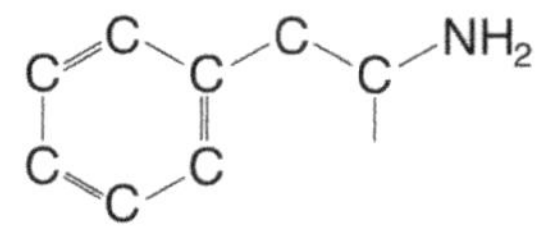

Fig. 4. Amphetamine. Fat-soluble, it spreads widely in the brain and heightens what I have called "generalized CNS arousal."

amphetamine and methylphenidate is to increase central dopamine and norepinephrine activity, which, importantly for ADHD, impacts executive and attentional function."[36] Amphetamine is among the "first-line therapies" for children, adolescents and adults with ADHD because of its greater efficacy.

Chemistry. Amphetamine's structure is a simple six-carbon ring with a side chain that features an amine group (a nitrogen attached to two hydrogens) (Fig. 4). Methamphetamine simply adds a methyl group (one carbon, three hydrogens) and can be made easily.

Brain mechanisms. Amphetamine's main mechanism of action in the brain is to increase synaptic extracellular dopamine and norepinephrine levels. Raising extracellular levels of these substances is accomplished by inhibiting proteins, so-called "transporters," which ferry dopamine and noradrenalin back into cells. The sudden spike in dopamine levels, caused by meth, is responsible for the euphoria that addicts seek to maintain.

Some of the most exciting research on the consequences of increased extracellular dopamine has been published by the Japanese neuroscientist Tadashi Isa at the Department of

---

[36] Faraone SV. (2018) The pharmacology of amphetamine and methylphenidate: Relevance to the neurobiology of attention-deficit/hyperactivity disorder and other psychiatric comorbidities. *Neurosci Biobehav Rev* **87**, 255–270.

Neuroscience at the University of Kyoto.[37] His lab used selective activation of dopaminergic neurons in the midbrain (the "ventral tegmental area"), dopaminergic neurons usually associated with behavioral reward, and determined the animals' attitudes toward risk. They were activated, and their axons projected to specific microregions of the frontal cortex of the experimental monkeys. In the ventral part of one specific activated microregion, monkeys selected responses that led to high amounts of reward but had a high risk of no reward at all. In the dorsal part of that same microregion, activation of the dopaminergic input led to choices with a low amount of reward but also with a low risk of no reward at all. Thus, the consequences of higher levels of extracellular dopamine as a result of amphetamine use would depend on the exact place in the frontal cortex where the dopamine level is elevated.

IX. 3,4-Methylenedioxymethamphetamine (MDMA)

3,4-Methylenedioxymethamphetamine (MDMA) is no ordinary drug. The DEA, the same agency that pursues Walter White — the meth cook — in *Breaking Bad*, wants everyone to stay away from it. In a long fact sheet, the DEA reminds us that MDMA is a Schedule I drug, "meaning it has a high potential for abuse, no currently accepted medical use in treatment in the U.S., and a lack of accepted safety for use under medical supervision."

MDMA comes in tablets sold as "Ecstasy," which can be swallowed, crushed, or snorted. These are frequently laced with other drugs such as ketamine, cocaine, and methamphetamine,

[37] Sasaki R, Ohta Y, Onoe H, *et al.* (2024). Balancing risk-return decisions by manipulating the mesofrontal circuits in primates. *Science* **383**(6678), 55–61.

so consumers can never be sure what they buy on the street. Also, other drugs are sometimes sold as MDMA, which can lead to overdose and even death. Because MDMA is a popular party drug, users usually take it along with alcohol and marijuana.

Basically, the drug causes changes in perception and increased sensitivity to touch. Users experience increased sexual arousal and a need for stimulation. Other effects (see below) include confusion, anxiety, and sleep problems. The DEA states that "users of MDMA experience many of the same risks as users of other stimulants such as cocaine and amphetamines," which can include increased heart rate and blood pressure. In high doses, MDMA can interfere with the body's ability to regulate temperature, possibly leading to liver, kidney, and cardiovascular system failure — and even death.

MDMA (Fig. 5) is made in labs and is primarily smuggled across the U.S. border from Canada and (to a lesser extent) the Netherlands. A small number of clandestine labs have been identified in the U.S.

MDMA gets into the brain easily because it is hydrophobic — it avoids water, but it interacts easily with the lipids (fats) in the brain. Current ideas about exactly how MDMA manages brain entry focus on a somewhat mysterious "transport protein," which now requires study. We note that MDMA can damage the

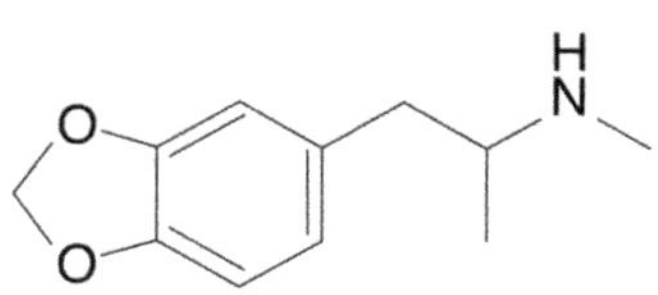

Fig. 5. MDMA. "Ecstasy." It can heighten sexual arousal and has a host of physiological effects. It binds to transporter proteins related to neurotransmitter functions: serotonin, dopamine, and norepinephrine.

blood–brain barrier, as shown by dye leakage. In the brain itself, MDMA can cause brain damage, as tracked by the growth and activation of glial cells (non-neuronal support cells) called "astrocytes."

In the brain, MDMA binds to proteins called "transporters" because of their ability to get neurotransmitters in and out of cells. For mechanisms of MDMA action in the brain, the transporter protein for the neurotransmitter serotonin is especially important; MDMA also binds to dopamine and norepinephrine transporters. These transporters work in both directions: to take a transmitter back up into the nerve cell, as well as to pump the transmitter out, affecting other nerve cells. Stanford professor Robert Malenka worked with genetically altered mice to show that MDMA works through the serotonin transporter in neurons at the serotonin transporter within the nucleus accumbens, a nerve cell group deep in the basal forebrain, to foster social approach.[38] In contrast, the rewarding properties of MDMA, likely supporting the effects on pleasure and euphoria, depend on dopamine receptors in nucleus accumbens neurons crucial for behavioral reinforcement.

As described by Sumit Sarkar and Larry Schmued, researchers at the Food and Drug Administration (FDA), "Ecstasy (MDMA) is a powerful hallucinogenic drug which has raised concern worldwide because of its high abuse liability."[39] These researchers have shown that "it also has the potential to produce degenerated neurons in discrete areas of the brain such as insular and parietal cortex, thalamus, and other specific brain regions." Neurons

---

[38] Rein B, Raymond K, Boustani C, *et al.* (2024) MDMA enhances empathy-like behaviors in mice via 5-HT release in the nucleus accumbens. *Sci Adv* **10**(17), eadl6554.

[39] Sarkar S & Schmued L (2010) Neurotoxicity of ecstasy (MDMA): An overview. *Curr Pharm Biotechnol* **11**(5), 460–469.

in the hippocampus came to their attention because of their role in regulating memory on the one hand and seizures on the other. Reduction of inhibitory neurons in the hippocampus was associated with an increase in susceptibility to seizures. Also, MDMA users performed significantly worse on immediate and delayed word recall tasks compared to non-users, highlighting that even low-frequency users are impacted by the drug. Neurotoxic effects of NMDA are most prominent in serotonergic systems. Psychiatric side effects following NMDA include depression. Further, Jessica Mead and Andrew Parrott at Swansea University in the U.K. documented a wide range of medical problems following MDMA use, even including fatalities.[40]

As noted, Ecstasy can cause neurotoxicity to the serotonergic system in the brain. This toxicity is linked to permanent physical and psychiatric problems. Undesirable acute psychological effects commonly reported during the drug experience include "hyperactivity, inability to focus one's thoughts in a sustained and useful manner, and insomnia. Related complaints often include mild hallucinations, depersonalization (a feeling of separation of the self from the body), emotional and personality problems, mental and behavioral problems, anxiety, agitation, and bizarre or reckless behavior. And impairment of memory, both verbal and visual." Effects that can also include impairment of decision-making ("executive function"), information processing, logical reasoning, and simple problem solving, occur even sometimes after the individual has stopped using MDMA. In certain cases, severe depression, which is sometimes resistant to any treatment other

---

[40] Mead J & Parrott A. (2020) Mephedrone and MDMA: A comparative review. *Brain Res* **1735**, 146740.

than selective serotonin reuptake inhibitors, is occasionally accompanied by suicidal thoughts.

Australian researchers Gordian Fulde and Lesley Forster have focused on the increase in production and availability of metamphetamines of note, according to Robert J. Sottile and Thomas Vida at the UNLV School of Medicine, because MDMA is associated primarily with raves, intoxication, and abuse.[41] As noted here, clinical findings reveal mental health and long-term neurological problems in persons taking or who have taken the drug. Because of these, "It is clear that the use of methamphetamine-type substances places an increasing burden on acute health services. There is a need for preventive and harm-minimization strategies."

Withdrawal by MDMA users causes relative deficits in mnemonic (memory loss) and executive functions (sometimes accompanied by intense fear). They can have extreme fatigue, low mood, and social withdrawal after stopping use.

X. Caffeine

In November 2023, two people died after drinking "charged lemonade" that contained nearly the same amount of caffeine as five 8-oz. cans of Red Bull. The incidents raised questions — and prompted a lawsuit — concerning the safety of so-called energy drinks spiked with high doses of caffeine. More generally, it renewed questions about how much caffeine is safe, since caffeine is a go-to source for stimulation throughout the day (and

---

[41] Sottile RJ & Vida T. (2022) A proposed mechanism for the MDMA-mediated extinction of traumatic memories in PTSD patients treated with MDMA-assisted therapy. *Front Psychiatry* **13**, 991753.

the source of billions of dollars of profit for companies promoting coffee and other specialty drinks that offer a "buzz").

Caffeine is a drug, even though most people wouldn't classify it as a stimulant like amphetamine and MDMA. As with many drugs, it is possible to develop a tolerance for caffeine (some people can drink six cups of coffee a day and barely feel the effects, while others get jumpy after only two). This is why people who started off with a few cups a day in college now need much more to stay "buzzed." But beyond the buzz, here are some other effects (cited by Australian health authorities) of too much caffeine:

- Increased body temperature
- Frequent urination
- Dehydration
- Dizziness
- Headaches
- Heart palpitations
- Restlessness, excitability, anxiety, and irritability
- Trembling hands
- Insomnia
- Tiredness after a brief energy spurt

Research suggests that to avoid most of these effects, a dosage of around 400 mg per day is generally acceptable, though this will vary depending on whether your body is used to regular doses of caffeine and how much you receive in a single dose. This works out to about three cups of coffee a day. So, if you're drinking coffee, it's important to read the labels on your other sources of caffeine if you want to stay within the limits that you can tolerate.

Chemically, what is caffeine?

Caffeine is a relatively simple organic compound: a so-called methylxanthine. Xanthine itself comprises 2 rings formed by carbon-to-carbon bonds and carbon-to-nitrogen bonds, and caffeine is distinguished by methyl groups (each with 1 carbon and 3 hydrogens) hooked to the nitrogens (Fig. 6). Caffeine crosses the blood–brain barrier; in fact, its receptors may regulate the blood–brain barrier. Once in the brain, its solubility in lipids (fats) allows it to diffuse easily. Its pharmacokinetics in the brain, measured in hours, are dominated by the enzyme CYP1A2, which metabolizes it. Depending on the individual, its effects can last up to 12 hours.

Caffeine interacts in the brain with adenosine receptors. Adenosine is a multi-use chemical that can be modified to provide one of the units of DNA. It can be joined with phosphate groups to perform crucial cellular signaling in the cytoplasm, and — most importantly for our purpose — it is a neuromodulator. It is a relatively large biochemical compared to others we have covered in this series, with a molecular weight of 267.

In the brain, the binding of adenosine to two of its receptors, A1 and A2a, is especially important neurophysiologically. Both these proteinaceous receptors (each has more than 300 amino acids) are on the neuronal and glial cell membrane; each crosses the membrane seven times, allowing for the formation of three

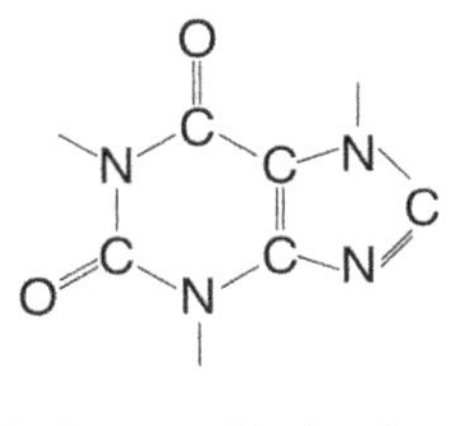

Fig. 6. Caffeine. In the brain, it blocks the adenosine A2a receptor.

extracellular loops and three intracellular loops. Both A1 and A2a are found throughout the brain. Experiments in transfected cells demonstrate the ability of A1 receptors to dimerize (2 chemicals joined) with A2a receptors, and the A1-A2a receptor dimer (compound of two receptors) can be biochemically identified in the striatum, in striatal glutamatergic terminals.

Background on adenosine: Purines and pyrimidines make up the two groups of nitrogen-containing chemicals (here "bases"), including the two groups of nucleotide bases: The purine bases are guanine (G) and adenine (A), each with two rings made from nine atoms. Purine bases also play an essential role in many metabolic and signaling processes within the compounds guanosine monophosphate (GMP) and adenosine monophosphate (AMP). Adenosine is adenine attached to ribose, a sugar.

Caffeine's actions to increase alertness and movement depend primarily on its blocking of the adenosine A2a receptor. Using this mechanism, adenosine can inhibit the release of neurotransmitters, reduce anxiety, act against convulsions, and reduce pain. Working through A2a, adenosine can reduce locomotor activity. The two receptors, A1 and A2a, work through different signaling systems in the cytoplasm.

In the brain, adenosine acts predominantly as an inhibitory neurotransmitter, working through A1 receptors. But, excitatory actions of adenosine, mediated by the activation of the A2a adenosine receptor subtype, have also been shown in the central nervous system. Furthermore, adenosine participates in so-called "tripartite synapses" (presynaptic neuron, postsynaptic neuron, astrocyte glial cell) as it is released from the astrocyte with the effect of suppressing the activity of other synapses. Thus, complexities abound: Adenosine can have different neurophysiological effects by working through different receptors. Some physiological effects of adenosine are mediated by its actions on other neurotransmitters. The tripartite synapse adds a layer of complexity. So, by extension, caffeine's actions in the brain take on the same complexities.

Caffeine intake has some potentially positive implications for human health. Some data support the contention that caffeine may "delay the onset of Parkinson's Disease in a dose-dependent manner." By blocking adenosine receptors, caffeine may militate against cognitive disturbances in the aged. Agonists of the A1 receptor have analgesic effects mediated not by classical binding but by indirect "allosteric" actions. All such studies have sparked commercial interest, e.g., coffee companies wanting to try out these agonists, with some initiatives reaching the stages of clinical trials.

Caffeine has also been shown to predispose individuals against developing cardiovascular disease and diabetes. Epidemiological data also suggest that habitual coffee consumption lowers the risk of Parkinson's and Alzheimer's disease, as well as a decreased risk of some cancers. Interpretation of the data on coffee must be conservative because coffee is a blend of hundreds of chemical compounds.

Quite separate from the potentially positive medical effects associated with caffeine, there are other things to worry about. For example, researchers worry about long-term or excessive caffeine consumption on sleep, migraine, and intraocular pressure. Further, long-term or over-consumption of caffeine can lead to addiction, insomnia, migraine, and other side effects. Withdrawal symptoms from caffeine addiction can include headaches and feelings of exhaustion.

Thus, as with so many drugs, consumers should weigh their positive and negative effects relative to their own, individual responses.

XI. Phencyclidine (PCP)

"Angel dust". Phencyclidine (aka PCP, from the formal name phenyl cyclohexyl piperidine) is an anesthetic that acts in the brain to produce a range of effects, including altered perception and hallucinations. Its use can also lead to psychosis. Transitions from recreational use to psychotic conditions such as schizophrenia have been reported. Schifano and Guirguis at the University of Hertfordshire note that "Phencyclidine, commonly known as 'angel dust,' induces analgesia in humans without rendering them unconscious; but with inducing amnesia, a phenomenon termed dissociative anesthesia" (dissociate the mind from the body).[42]

PCP can be taken in the form of a dry powder or smoked, with cigarettes sometimes dipped in a solution of PCP dissolved in an organic solvent (Fig. 7). A PCP overdose can trigger agitation, intense emotional releases, hallucinations, and psychosis. In severe cases, it can lead to seizures, coma, hyperthermia, and muscular rigidity.

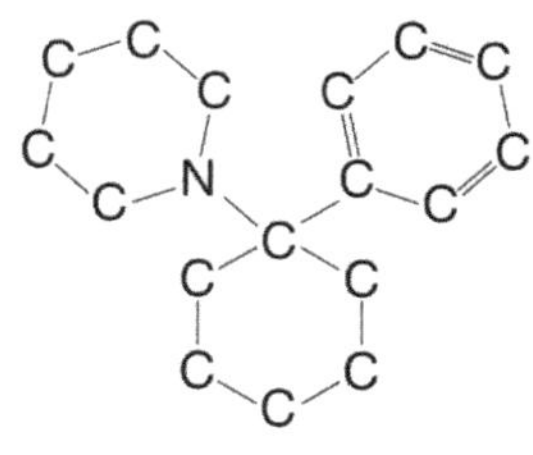

Fig. 7. Phencyclidine (PCP). "Angel dust." An anesthetic, it can alter perception.

[42] Schifano F, Chiappini S, Corkery JM, *et al.* (2021) The e-psychonaut drugs' psychopharmacology. *Curr Opin Pharmacol* **57**, 165–174.

Its actions begin within minutes and last for hours. Its lipid (fat) solubility allows it to spread widely in the lipid-rich brain and cross the blood–brain barrier. As a street drug, used for recreation, PCP is consumed for its mind-altering effects and, under some conditions, for inducing euphoria. But in addition to risking seizures and coma, as noted, users may in some cases also risk addiction.

Mechanisms

PCP works by blocking one type of receptor for the neurotransmitter glutamate, the NMDA receptor, a complex receptor with multiple modes of action. By inhibiting NMDA receptors, PCP disrupts perception, various thought processes, and motor controls. Most severely, PCP can cause a "dissociation from reality," i.e., delusions.

Metabolites

An authoritative review from the lab of Professor Gabriele Sani deals with PCP metabolite, 3-Methoxy-Phencyclidine (3-MeO-PCP), another non-competitive antagonist of glutamate NMDA receptors. This compound does not yet have great recreational interest, but nevertheless gets attention for "its extremely toxic, sometimes fatal, effects." 3-MeO-PCP can cause "erratic behavior, confusion, disorientation, dissociation, hallucinations, and other signs of psychosis, often associated with altered neurological status and amnesia."[43]

---

[43] Pepe M, Di Nicola M, Cocciolillo F, *et al.* (2024) 3-methoxy-phencyclidine induced psychotic disorder: A literature review and an ^{18}F-FDG PET/CT case report. *Pharmaceuticals (Basel)* **17**(4), 452.

Romain Pelletier, at the University of Rennes, observes that PCP (and its metabolites) had its heyday in 1976, with many newspaper and television reports on its recreational use.[44] "Despite stricter law enforcement controls, a move to Schedule II of the United States' Controlled Substances Act in January 1978 and a fall in media coverage, consumption of PCP has been increasing steadily after a slight decline in the late 1980s."

Another PCP-like compound metabolite is ketamine (see above). Ketamine can serve as an analgesic and a "dissociative" sedative that produces potent analgesia. It is rapidly gaining acceptance in the management of pain. Liang Zhou and Jingjing Duan, in Suzhou, China, have documented that both the anesthetic and antidepressant effects of ketamine are mediated by N-methyl-D-aspartate receptor (NMDAR) inhibition.[45]

PCP and its metabolites are party drugs. Tomohisa Mori and Tsutomu Suzuki write that "Over the past two decades, patterns of drug abuse have changed, so that club/recreational drugs such as PCP, MDMA, ketamine, and synthetic cannabinoids, which induce perceptual distortions, like hallucinations, are now more commonly abused, especially by young people."[46] The desired effects are euphoria, a feeling of intimacy, altered visual perception, enhanced libido, and increased energy. Caroline Copeland

---

[44] Pelletier R, Le Daré B, Grandin L, *et al.* (2022) New psychoactive substance cocktail in an intensive care intoxication case elucidated by molecular networking. *Clin Toxicol (Phila)* **60**(1), 122–125.

[45] Zhou L & Duan G. (2024) The role of NMDARs in the anesthetic and antidepressant effects of ketamine. *CNS Neurosci Therapeut* **30**(4), e14464.

[46] Mori T & Suzuki T. (2018) The discriminative stimulus properties of hallucinogenic and dissociative anesthetic drugs. *Curr Top Behav Neurosci* **39**, 141–152.

and her team at King's College London detailed the first fatality due to 3-MeO-PCP intoxication to be reported in the U.K. "Users of 3-MeO-PCP should be cautioned against its use as a club drug or in a similar setting where elevations in heart rate, body temperature, and blood pressure may occur."[47]

Schizophrenia-like episodes

As Okubo, Okada, and Motomura have observed, the widely espoused "dopamine hypothesis for the pathophysiology of schizophrenia" (saying, roughly, that the disease follows from a dopamine overload) can now be joined by a "glutamate hypothesis" based on clinical findings that NMDAR antagonists, such as PCP induce schizophrenia-like psychotic episodes.[48]

PCP disrupts hippocampal electrical activity in such a manner that exaggerates long-term synaptic depression. This neural discoordination could be central to varied cognitive and sensorimotor impairments.

Rachel Hill's lab at Monash University studied how NMDAR antagonists like PCP cause psychosis-like symptoms by working with mice, where such symptoms include hyperlocomotion.[49] The effect of hyperlocomotion is negated in mice in which a particular

---

[47] Copeland CS, Hudson S, Treble R, & Hamnett HJ. (2022) The first fatal intoxication with 3-MeO-PCP in the UK and a review of the literature, *J Anal Toxicol* **46**(5), 461–470.

[48] Okubo R, Okada M, & Motomura E. (2024) Dysfunction of the NMDA receptor in the pathophysiology of schizophrenia and/or the pathomechanisms of treatment-resistant schizophrenia, *Biomolecules* **14**(9), 1128.

[49] Vinnakota C, Hudson MR, Ikeda K, *et al.* (2025) Effects of NMDA receptor antagonists on working memory and gamma oscillations, and the mediating role of the GluN2D subunit. *Neuropsychopharmacology*.

subunit of the NMDAR (GluN2D) has been genetically knocked out. This result demonstrates how, on the one hand, it will be necessary to identify the contributions of separate elements of the receptor to achieve a complete understanding of PCP mechanisms. On the other hand, we must also envision what Rockefeller University's Roderick MacKinnon has called "higher order transient" structures involved in membrane signaling, relations among membrane proteins that can be formed and reformed usefully.[50] In summary, although the temporary pleasure from PCP and its metabolites is well-known, the dangers must be acknowledged and emphasized.

XII. Barbiturates

Chemistry. Barbituric acid is a simple 6-member ring — 4 carbons and 2 nitrogens — oxygens attached, with perfect left/right symmetry.

According to the DEA, barbiturates can be used as "sedatives, hypnotics, anesthetics, and anticonvulsants." They reduce excitation in the central nervous system.

Abuse. However, overdoses can reduce the depth of respiration and weaken the pulse. Patients can become dependent on barbiturates. They will use some barbiturates in a manner that leads to intoxication and mood changes (a "high" or "buzz"), followed by dependence and addiction. Further, there is the danger of coma and even death. So, this is yet another drug whose beneficial uses must be weighed against its potential harm when used indiscriminately.

---

[50] Zhang Y, Mazal H, Mandala VS, *et al*. (2025) Higher-order transient membrane protein structures. *Proc Nat Acad Sci* **122**(1), e2421275121.

Several uses

Migraines. The lab of Daniele Martinelli at the University of Pavia studies how to use barbiturates to treat migraine attacks.[51] They favor a stratified approach: when dealing with severe attacks and after initial treatment with a drug that acts through serotonin receptors, they turn to barbiturates. In contrast, Dimos Mitsikostas at the University of Athens emphasized that instead of using barbiturates to relieve certain symptoms, there could be a range of approaches, including serotonergic drugs designed specifically for migraine, as well as aspirin, ibuprofen, naproxen, and transcranial magnetic stimulation.[52]

Anxiety. The literature offers proof that barbiturates can be used to reduce anxiety, serve as anticonvulsants (i.e., fighting seizures), and help people get to sleep. They increase the total sleep time, decrease sleep latency, and decrease the number of awakenings during the night.

Epilepsy. Alexander Bryson and Robert Richardson at the Florey Institute of Neuroscience and Mental Health, in Melbourne, have concentrated on the long-term management of epilepsy. They state that: "In addition to older medications (like barbiturates) that have well-defined roles for the treatment of epilepsy, recent discoveries into the structure and function of the $GABA_A$ receptor (see below) have led to the development of newer compounds designed to maximise therapeutic benefit whilst minimising adverse effects." At the Universite Libre de Bruselles, Nicolas Gaspard emphasizes the use of continuous

---

[51] Martinelli D, Pocora MM, & Tassorelli C. (2024) Nonspecific analgesics, combination analgesics, and antiemetics. *Handb Clin Neurol* **199**, 3–16.

[52] Mitsikostas DD & Ward TN. (2024) Evidence-based symptomatic treatment of migraine. *Handb Clin Neurol* **199**, 203–218.

video electroencephalogram (EEG) to battle stubborn hard-to-reverse epilepsy, called "super-refractory status epilepticus."[53]

End of life. Finally, barbiturates in high doses can be used for medical assistance in dying.

Mechanisms

Barbiturates act throughout the brain. They work by making GABA receptors (Fig. 8), which are inhibitory in the sense that they reduce neuronal signaling and operate more efficiently. They enhance the flow of the negative chloride ions through the pore in the GABA receptor to reduce the ability of the neuron to fire off an action potential. Barbiturates are so-called "allosteric modulators," which means that instead of simply blocking the GABA binding site, they act at molecular sites some distance from the binding site, among the complex receptor components.

GABA receptors are complicated. As elucidated by Scott M. Thompson at the University of Colorado School of Medicine, these receptors have three types of components: alphas, betas, and gammas.[54] There are 6 types of alphas; 3 types of betas and 3 types of gammas. On any given nerve cell, there may be receptors with 2 alphas, 2 betas, and 1 gamma. Looking at the full GABA receptor from just outside the nerve cell membrane, there is symmetry with

---

[53] Richardson RJ, Petrou S, & Bryson A. (2024) Established and emerging $GABA_A$ receptor pharmacotherapy for epilepsy. *Front Pharmacol* **15**, 1341472; Rossetti AO, Claassen J, & Gaspard N. (2024) Status epilepticus in the ICU. *Intensive Care Med* **50**(1), 1–16.

[54] Thompson SM. (2024) Modulators of GABA(A) receptor-mediated inhibition in the treatment of neuropsychiatric disorders: Past, present, and future. *Neuropsychopharmacology* **49**(1), 83–95.

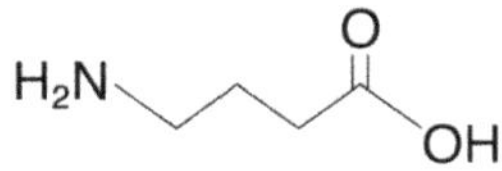

Fig. 8. GABA (re barbiturates). GABA is an inhibitory neurotransmitter in the sense that it reduces neuronal signaling.

an alpha on each side, a beta on each side, all around a gamma. Barbiturates bind near the transmembrane interfaces of β subunits with α or γ subunits.

Surprisingly, barbiturates can directly open $GABA_A$ receptor channels in the absence of GABA. Barbiturates increase the time that channels remain open in response to a fixed concentration of GABA, whereas benzodiazepines (chemicals often used for similar purposes) increase channel opening frequency.

Although barbiturates have been around for a long time, they are still subjects of active research, both to improve their effectiveness and to reduce harmful side effects.

XIII. Benzodiazepines

According to the DEA, benzodiazepines "are depressants that produce sedation and hypnosis, relieve anxiety and reduce seizures." Unfortunately, they can also produce amnesia and irritability, and following high doses, lightheadedness and even delirium.

Benzodiazepine abuse includes intentional overdosage to the point of addiction. Their use as "party drugs" is not thought to be frequent, but when they are, it seems to be to induce euphoria.

Their chemistry features three rings of carbon and nitrogen atoms with a composition of $C_{16}H_{11}ClN_2O_3$, and a molecular weight of around 315 (Fig. 9). The chemical structures do not look like those of barbiturates, even though some of the mental effects are like those of barbiturates.

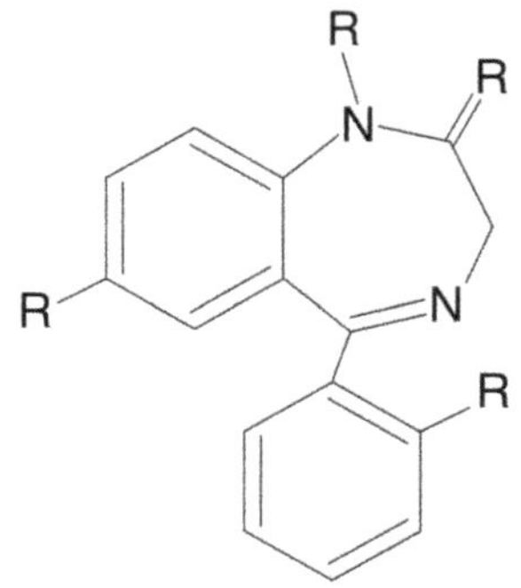

Fig. 9. Benzodiazepines. Have long been used to produce sedation and hypnosis and to relieve anxiety.

Uses

Anxiety disorders are the most diagnosed psychiatric pathology. Yet while the costs to society are substantial, existing treatments are often inadequate. Benzodiazepines possess remarkable anxiolytic efficacy, reducing anxiety, but they have fallen out of favor due to adverse effects that include unintended sedation, motor impairment, addictive potential, and tolerance development. Accordingly, there has been a substantial effort to design other benzodiazepine-like anxiolytics with reduced sedative liabilities.

Ingrid Y. Liu's lab in Taiwan has focused on the use of diazepines to aid healthful sleep; thus, to reduce insomnia. Recently, she stated that "Good sleep quality helps promote the performance of daily functions. In contrast, insufficient sleep reduces the efficiency of daily activities and increases the risk of having accidents. Several studies emphasized that dysfunction of the GABAergic system is related to insomnia, the most prevalent sleep-related disorder."[55]

---

[55] Varinthra P, Anwar SNMN, Shih S-C, & Liu IY. (2024) The role of the GABAergic system on insomnia. *Tzu Chi Med J* **36**(2), 103–109.

Universally, researchers focus on the inhibitory GABAergic system to reduce insomnia. Benzodiazepines reduce sleep latency. Thus, among other approaches, benzodiazepines are viewed as a primary approach to fostering healthful sleep. In this regard, Dinesh Pal and his colleagues at the University of Michigan used benzodiazepine compounds to sedate experimental rats for EEG studies of recovery and sleep homeostasis.[56]

There are issues surrounding the use of GABA enhancers like benzodiazepines, which play a significant role in behavioral medicine, and there are side effects that limit their use. In addition, there is a lack of clarity of concept, for example, with respect to discrete anxiety disorders, e.g., which benzodiazepine should be chosen for which type of anxiety disorder? We need a better understanding of receptor-related actions and neurobiological mechanisms associated with anxiety.

Bryson and Richardson, at the Florey Institute of Neuroscience and Mental Health at the University of Melbourne, reviewed the use of benzodiazepines in "clinical practice for both the long-term management of epilepsy and emergency seizure control." They concentrate on the "development of newer compounds designed to maximise therapeutic benefit whilst minimising adverse effects" while predicting that "drugs that modulate the $GABA_A$ receptor will remain a cornerstone of epilepsy management for the foreseeable future."

Mechanisms

Benzodiazepines work by making GABA receptors, which are inhibitory in the sense that they reduce neuronal signaling, work

[56] Silverstein BH, Parkar A, Groenhout T, *et al.* (2024) Effect of prolonged sedation with dexmedetomidine, midazolam, propofol, and sevoflurane on sleep homeostasis in rats. *Br J Anaesth* **132**(6), 1248–1259.

more efficiently. Benzodiazepines are so-called "allosteric modulators," which means that instead of simply blocking the GABA binding site, they act at molecular sites some distance from the binding site among the complex receptor components. The bottom line is that, because of benzodiazepine action, more chloride ions flow through the receptors' pores, making the cell more negative and reducing signaling by action potentials.

As noted above, and with regard to barbiturates, GABA receptors are complicated. GABA receptors have three types of components: alphas, betas, and gammas. There are 6 types of alphas: 3 types of betas and 3 types of gammas. On any given nerve cell, there will be receptors with 2 alphas, 2 betas, and 1 gamma. Looking at the full GABA receptor from just outside the nerve cell membrane, you will be able to see symmetry, with an alpha on each side, a beta on each side, and all around a gamma.

Benzodiazepines potentiate GABA receptors containing gamma-2 subunits. This is because they bind at the interface of gamma-2 and an alpha subunit. In the brain, the predominant GABA receptor isoform is Alpha-1, Beta-2, and Gamma-2. Most experts would say that a high-affinity binding site for benzodiazepines is located at the α/γ subunit interface in the extracellular domain of the $GABA_A$ receptor.

In the alpha-1 subunit of the GABA receptor, activity requires the amino acid histidine at a specific position in the receptor protein — a mutation that abolishes histidine leaves the receptor insensitive to benzodiazepine. Functionally, benzodiazepines increase channel opening frequency, whereas barbiturates increase the time that GABA receptor channels remain open in response to a fixed concentration of GABA.

Ryan E. Hibbs' lab at the University of Texas Southwestern used cryo-electron microscopy to determine the structure of a human synaptic GABA receptor.[57] The occupied benzodiazepine site was observed at the single $\alpha 1$-$\gamma 2$ interface. Surprising results revealed two distinct transmembrane domain conformations (i.e., shapes of the GABA receptor protein), the meaning of which is obscure.

In general, different alpha subunits are thought to be responsible for different medical uses: sedative, anxiolytic, anticonvulsant, muscle-relaxing, and pain-relieving uses.

Cerne and Lippa, at the Laboratory of Antiepileptic Drug Discovery in Indianapolis, have been working to replace conventional benzodiazepines because of safety and tolerability concerns, as well as side effects that include motor impairment and respiratory depression.[58] One specific class of candidates to replace benzodiazepines is surprising: a small group of steroid hormones called "neuroactive steroids." Trials are ongoing.

Benzodiazepine withdrawal is widely known to cause a variety of symptoms: nausea, tremors, postural hypotension, malaise, psychomotor agitation, anxiety, insomnia, irritability, palpitations, headache, hallucinations, seizures, and delirium. Effective withdrawal can be achieved by tapering off the dose, as an outpatient, if possible; otherwise, with inpatient withdrawal at a hospital.

In summary, this broad class of GABA receptor modulators has been proven useful for medical conditions, but still generates new research with the aim of improving the benefit/side effect ratio.

XIV. Alcohol

Ethanol (alcohol) is a very simple chemical with a molecular weight of only 46. It features a backbone of 2 carbon atoms, surrounded

---

[57] Kim JJ & Hibbs RE. (2021) Direct structural insights into GABA(A) receptor pharmacology. *Trends Biochem Sci* **46**(6), 502–517.

[58] Cerne R, Smith JL, Chrzanowska A, & Lippa A. (2024) Nonsedating anxiolytics. *Pharmacol Biochem Behav* **245**, 173895.

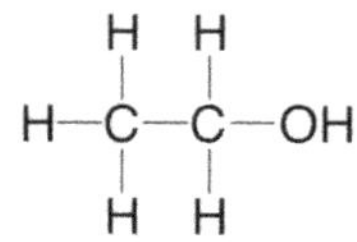

Fig. 10. Ethanol (alcohol) use by humans in history goes all the way back to the ancient Mesopotamian city of Ur, 10,000 years ago.

by 6 hydrogen atoms and 1 oxygen (Fig. 10). It is widely distributed in the brain.

While alcohol has long been used for relaxation and sociality, it has always been associated with dangerous behavior. Recently, it has been linked to cancer. It is acknowledged to be abused, and it can become addictive.

Mechanisms

The inhibitory actions of the neurotransmitter GABA — actions that will reduce activity in the neuron that receives the GABA — are a big story here. In the words of Professor Esa Korpi, in Helsinki, "The target of alcohol's effect on the central nervous system has been sought for more than 50 years in the brain's GABA system."[59] Indeed, $GABA_A$ receptors have been shown to be one of the sites of alcohol's action. Even extremely low concentrations of ethanol can potentiate the function of GABA receptors if they are made of certain specific "alpha, beta, and gamma" subunits.

The molecular mechanisms of GABAergic inhibition have been a hotspot of research, but Professor Korpi reflects that they "have turned out to be complex and controversial." More work needs to be done.

---

[59] Korpi ER & Sinkkonen ST. (2006) GABA(A) receptor subtypes as targets for neuropsychiatric drug development. *Pharmacol Ther* **109**(1–2), 12–32.

Most research on the connection between alcohol and GABA has been performed using nerve cells. But Professor Doo-Sup Choi, at the Mayo Clinic, has discovered that astrocytes can also synthesize and release GABA, activating GABA receptors in neighboring neurons in normal physiological and pathological conditions. As the primary homeostatic glial cells in the brain, astrocytes play a crucial role in regulating GABA homeostasis and synaptic neurotransmission. Choi posits that astrocytic GABA dysregulation may be implicated in psychiatric disorders, such as major depressive disorder.[60]

Some research on alcohol-related behaviors has taken a genetic turn. For example, a genome-wide associated study compared the alcoholic drinks per week and pathological drinking behaviors to controls. It charted genomic differences and, importantly, DNA methylation sites. The authors identified 10 alcohol-related CpG DNA methylation sites on the DNA, where a methyl group, a carbon atom, and 3 hydrogen atoms have been attached, and believed that these were causally related to psychiatric disorders.

An authoritative report from the laboratory of Professor Rainer Spanagel in Mannheim, looked for genetic differences between alcohol-dependent subjects and controls.[61] The study, which included humans, monkeys, and rodents, analyzed gene expression in the PFC (crucial for cognitive performance), nucleus accumbens (activity related to behavioral reward), and the amygdala (regulating emotional state). The PFC had

---

[60] Ali DN, Ali HM, Lopez MR, *et al.* (2024) Astrocytic gabaergic regulation in alcohol use and major depressive disorders. *Cells* **13**(4), 318.

[61] Spanagel R. (2020) Cannabinoids and the endocannabinoid system in reward processing and addiction: From mechanisms to interventions. *Dialogues Clin Neurosci* **22**(3), 241–250.

the highest number of differentially expressed genes (alcohol-dependent vs. control subjects), featuring genes for enzymes, which add phosphates to other proteins, as well as a transcription factor (turns on gene expression) related to immune responses. This impressively comprehensive study does not boil down to a simple, single "story."

Professor Nihal Salem at the University of Texas observes that the PFC is a crucial regulator of alcohol dependence.[62] Comparing alcohol-dependent animals to controls, his team performed single-nucleus RNA sequencing and gene expression profiling on cells of the medial prefrontal cortex. He states: "A subtype of inhibitory neurons was the most alcohol-sensitive cell type and contained a downregulated gene co-expression module; the hub gene for this module is Cpa6, a gene previously identified by genetic studies to be associated with excessive alcohol consumption." This gene codes for an enzyme that works on proteins and is widely expressed in the brain. These interesting findings were not limited to neurons: Genetic differences between alcohol-dependent and control animals were also discovered in astrocytes and microglia.

Professor Mitra Sadat-Shirazi, at Tufts, focused on potential effects of alcohol on epigenetic (meaning "beyond" genetic) mechanisms, including DNA methylation and modification of histone proteins coating the DNA.[63] Alcohol has the capability to induce changes in the epigenome, the network of enzymes and other

---

[62] Salem NA, Manzano L, Keist MW, *et al.* (2024) Cell-type brain-region specific changes in prefrontal cortex of a mouse model of alcohol dependence. *Neurobiol Dis* **190**, 106361.

[63] Heidari NN, Hajikarim-Hamedani A, Heidari A, *et al.* (2024) Alcohol: Epigenome alteration and inter/transgenerational effect. *Alcohol* **117**, 27–41.

proteins that regulate access to DNA. The most extensive research has highlighted alcohol-induced changes in DNA methylation, a chemical process associated with inhibition of gene transcription (gene expression that makes a new RNA, thus to achieve synthesis of a new protein), but there have also been reports of modifications of chemical reactions that add acetyl groups to the histone proteins, which coat the DNA. Notably, rodent studies suggest that these epigenetic changes can result in lasting phenotype (bodily) alterations that extend across at least two generations.

There is confusion about acute versus chronic alcohol consumption. One review concluded that acute and chronic alcohol exposure can induce opposite modifications in epigenetic mechanisms: acute alcohol exposure increases histone acetylation, decreases histone methylation, and inhibits DNA methyltransferase activity, while chronic alcohol exposure induces hypermethylation of DNA.

A completely different path to the analysis of alcohol's actions was taken by Professor Fan Yang at Xinxiang Medical University. This team focused on the effects of alcohol on certain basic components of cells, namely sphingolipids.[64] These fatty molecules are lipids based on a sphingosine backbone, and are essential components of cell membranes. They are abundant in the brain. Sphingosine is an 18-carbon amino alcohol with a hydrocarbon chain, which forms a primary part of sphingolipids, a class of cell membrane lipids that can mediate but cause inflammation in the brain. This is a difficult area of study because different sphingolipids may have different effects on alcohol use disorder.

---

[64] Wang C, Yan J, Du K, *et al.* (2023) Intestinal microbiome dysbiosis in alcohol-dependent patients and its effect on rat behaviors. *mBio* **14**(6), e0239223.

Professor Elisabet Jerlhag at the University of Gothenburg takes another approach to studying alcohol. She writes that peptides, small pieces of proteins, of the gut–brain axis "have gained recent attention as potential treatment targets for addiction."[65] While the number of gut–brain peptides is vast, the gut peptide ghrelin and glucagon-like peptide-1 (GLP-1) have been suggested as important players. Ghrelin is traditionally considered a peptide that encourages eating through its actions in the hypothalamus, but "recent studies found that it increases alcohol intake in rodents and craving for alcohol in humans." The opposite kind of experiment, a suppression of the ghrelin receptor, attenuated alcohol-related responses in animals.

During attempts at withdrawal after regular drinking, patients may, several hours after the last drink, note increased blood pressure, increased body temperature, tremor, insomnia, anxiety, nausea, vomiting, and/or headache.

In summary, alcohol is deeply involved with the biochemistry of the brain in several different ways.

XV. Nicotine

Nicotine is a small organic chemical featuring two rings of carbon and nitrogen (Fig. 11). It is inhaled through smoking or vaping and is classified as a stimulant. As such, it can enhance the performance of tasks that require alertness and attention, as well as some aspects of motoric function. It is highly addictive.

In the brain, nicotine works through a class of protein receptors for the neurotransmitter acetylcholine. As reviewed thoroughly by

---

[65] Jerlhag E. (2025) GLP-1 receptor agonists: Promising therapeutic targets for alcohol use disorder. *Endocrinology* **166**(4), bqaf028.

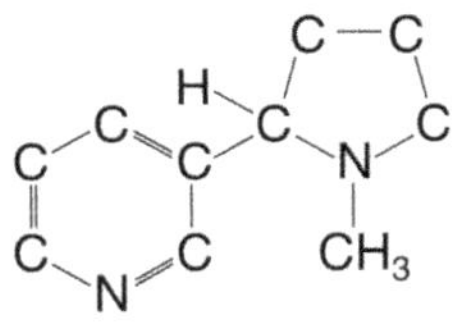

Fig. 11. Nicotine can enhance alertness and attention. It works by binding to nicotinic acetylcholine receptors in the brain (Fig. 12).

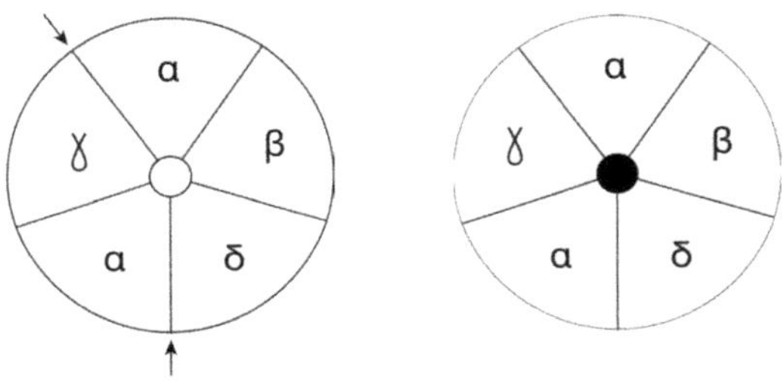

Fig. 12. Nicotinic acetylcholine receptors. Composed of five proteins here, identified by Greek letters. The open receptor (left) shows sites (arrows) where nicotine can bind. Ions, like sodium or calcium, can flow through the open central pore. The closed receptor (right) shows (black circle) the central pore closed following an alteration of proteins' conformations.

Ruthie E. Wittenberg working with John Dani in the Department of Neuroscience at the University of Pennsylvania, nicotine binds to so-called "nicotinic" acetylcholine receptors (Fig. 12) that are widespread in the brain.[66] Each receptor is composed of five proteins, each of which spans the nerve cell membrane four times; the five proteins are arranged symmetrically around a pore. Nicotine binds at an interface between two of these five proteins, at which time the conformations of all five proteins change, opening a channel through which positively charged ions, like sodium, potassium,

[66] Wittenberg RE, Wolfman SL, De Biasi M, & Dani JA, *et el.* (2020) Nicotinic acetylcholine receptors and nicotine addiction: A brief introduction. *Neuropharmacology* **177**, 108256.

or calcium, can flow. That ionic flow "excites" the nerve cell, meaning that the rate of electrical firing, or signaling, by that cell will increase. When this happens in a dopamine neuron, which projects its axon to the basal forebrain's nucleus accumbens, the smoker will feel a reward leading to potential addiction, as reviewed by the Damaj lab at Virginia Commonwealth University.[67]

Nicotinic acetylcholine receptors feature a wide variety of subtypes, leading to a wide range of physiological and pharmacological properties. This heterogeneity, coupled with the many phenomena following so-called "desensitization" of the receptors, i.e., a reduction of their effectiveness, renders this scientific field complex. However, it also creates molecular complexity, which could explain various aspects of nicotine's psychological effects; for example, a positive feeling (on the one hand) or depression (on the other). Of course, reward and depression are inconsistent with each other (see further below), which demonstrates the complexity of nicotine's effect on the brain and, hence, the complexity of this field of study.

In sum, as skillfully reviewed by Marina Picciotto at Yale's Department of Psychiatry, addiction to tobacco depends on members of the nicotinic acetylcholine receptor family, which are ligand-gated (nicotine-dependent) ion channels that form pentamers — 5-sided placements — arranged around a water-filled pore and allow for the influx of both Na+, K+, and Ca^{2+}.[68]

Brain regions and neural circuitry. Nicotine affects subpopulations of dopamine neurons differently, depending on where

---

[67] Muldoon PP, Lichtman AH, Parsons LH, & Damaj MI. (2013) The role of fatty acid amide hydrolase inhibition in nicotine reward and dependence. *Life Sci* **92**(8–9), 458–462.

[68] Picciotto MR & Kenny PJ. (2021) Mechanisms of nicotine addiction. *Cold Spring Harb Perspect Med* **11**(5), a039610.

their axons project. That is, nicotine excites neurons that project into the nucleus accumbens, which provides the feeling of reward. But nicotine also inhibits neurons that project into the amygdala nuclei and foster anxiety, as shown by Claire Nguyen working with Philippe Faure at ESPC in Paris.[69] We usually think of the amygdala as helping us identify and avoid sources of harm, but nicotine cravings seem to interfere with these functions. Amygdala neurons receive strong acetylcholine inputs, which work in part through nicotinic receptors. Blocking nicotinic receptors specifically in the amygdala can reduce "depressant-like" behaviors in experimental animals. Reviewers of the effects of nicotinic acetylcholine receptors in the amygdala describe them as "complex."

Nicotine acts through hippocampal circuits as well. When activated, nicotinic acetylcholine circuits located there cause increased depression- and anxiety-like behaviors in mice, reversible by blocking nicotinic receptors. Zubin Bhagwagar's lab linked nicotinic receptor dysfunction to major depressive disorders.[70] Another complex feature of this field is that a "stimulant," nicotine, can have actions that are associated with depression.

In the cerebral cortex, nicotinic cholinergic receptors contribute to the maintenance of attention, but the highest levels of cholinergic signaling can lead to psychiatric illness.

Genetics. Twin studies in which monozygotic ("identical") twins have a much higher concordance rate in nicotine addiction than dizygotic ("fraternal") twins show that genetics plays some

---

[69] Nguyen C, Mondoloni S, Le Borgne T, *et al.* (2021) Nicotine inhibits the VTA-to-amygdala dopamine pathway to promote anxiety. *Neuron* **109**(16), 2604–2615.e9.

[70] Saricicek A, Esterlis I, Maloney KH, *et al.* (2012) Persistent beta2-nicotinic acetylcholinergic receptor dysfunction in major depressive disorder. *Am J Psychiatry* **169**(8), 851–859.

role in the addiction. That's simple. But few simple answers have yet emerged regarding which individual genes are involved and the nature of their involvement.

Effects of smoking. As noted regarding nicotine dependence, specific members of the family of nicotinic receptors act in the reward-critical ventral tegmental brain area and terminals in the nucleus accumbens. When nicotine activates its receptors in this neuronal cell group, the well-studied dopaminergic reward mechanism reinforces nicotine use and, hence, smoking.

Though we tend to think of the physical effects of smoking, e.g., lung disease and cancer, it can also be deleterious to a smoker's mental state, causing depression. In this regard, while a smoker may not notice the slow creep of emphysema for years, he or she may notice a degraded mood fairly quickly. Thus, while it is notoriously hard to persuade people that (eventually) they could die from smoking, it may be easier to convince them to stop once they realize smoking's depressive effects. Ads advising people to stop smoking should play up these effects and remind people that if they are feeling dispirited, it may be the result of a habit they should kick.

Most attempts to stop smoking fail. This failure can be named "nicotine dependence." In the U.K., Paul Aveyard and Robert West at the University of Birmingham say that the rate of those trying to quit is high: 78 attempts per 100 smokers per year.[71] Nicotine-addicted smokers who do quit see that attentional and cognitive abilities are impaired, and their body weight increases. Many will get depressed. Medications that can help with withdrawal include Nicorette gum, nicotine patches, and nicotine

[71] Aveyard P & West R. (2007) Managing smoking cessation. *BMJ* **335**(7609), 37–41.

nasal spray. Therapeutic behavioral support is also useful. Relapse during or after treatment is common, and treatment for helping with withdrawal may be needed several times.

Late-breaking: Some recent work from the Mourot lab in Paris has raised hope for a high-tech approach to helping smokers stop smoking.[72] It turns out that neurons in the interpeduncular nucleus (IPN, a nerve cell group between the hypothalamus and the midbrain) respond to nicotine, and, by responding, the IPN neurons lower the rewarding effect of nicotine. Thus, we can foresee that high-tech microstimulation of IPN neurons should be therapeutically useful.

XVI. Anabolic Androgenic Steroids

Here are three definitions that help explain the structure and function of anabolic androgenic steroids (AAS) like testosterone:

- Anabolic: Promotes metabolic activity concerning biosynthesis of complex tissue (mainly muscle).
- Androgenic: Promotes male characteristics.
- Steroid: Carbon atoms distributed into four linked rings, which have various side groups whose chemical nature determines the type of individual steroid (among many).

So, in effect, compounds labeled "Anabolic androgenic steroids" are manufactured forms of testosterone, often given to men to promote male physiological characteristics, where these are

---

[72] Mondoloni S, Nguyen C, Vicq E, *et al.* (2023) Prolonged nicotine exposure reduces aversion to the drug in mice by altering nicotinic transmission in the interpeduncular nucleus. *Elife* **12**, e80767.

underdeveloped or in decline. They are also taken by men, usually in the absence of medical supervision, to enhance male characteristics. Since testosterone is fat-soluble, it can be widely distributed in the brain.

The DEA states that testosterone and several closely related steroids "promote muscle growth, enhance athletic and other physical performance and improve physical appearance." These may be desirable outcomes under medical supervision. But when not taken under medical supervision, as is frequently the case, the effects may be harmful.

Useful

Among the potentially useful effects of anabolic steroids are "body and performance enhancement" according to a 2024 review by Channa Jayasena and his team at Imperial College, London.[73] For example, a landmark study by Bhasin and collaborators in the 1990s showed that, without question, supraphysiological levels of administered testosterone increased muscle mass and strength in healthy men.[74]

Supraphysiological androgen administration can have a direct effect on men's behavior. In one study, participants reported euphoria, increased energy, and increased sexual arousal. But be careful: one subject experienced an acute manic episode during the study.

---

[73] Sharma A, Grant B, Islam H, *et al.* (2022) Common symptoms associated with usage and cessation of anabolic androgenic steroids in men. *Best Pract Res Clin Endocrinol Metab* **36**(5), 101691.

[74] Bhasin S, Krishnan V, Storer TW, *et al.* (2023) Androgens and selective androgen receptor modulators to treat functional limitations associated with aging and chronic disease. *J Gerontol A Biol Sci Med Sci* **78**(Supplement_1), 25–31.

Other studies have found no significant behavioral changes during supraphysiological testosterone administration in healthy men. In addition, not all androgenic hormones have the same effects.

Harm. Anabolic steroids can cause high blood pressure, cardiac abnormalities, high cholesterol, and acne, especially when the steroids are taken without medical supervision. Behavioral steroidal effects are complicated, but can include irritability, impulsivity, cognitive impairment, and reduced libido. Possible effects on aggressive behaviors are controversial and will be discussed separately.

The evolving prevalence of AAS abuse among nonathletes is alarming because of the known harm to an individual's health. Among the adverse effects of AAS abuse, male infertility and sexual dysfunction have often been reported in the literature. One study has shown that all-cause mortality is about two times higher in AAS abusers compared to a control group. Since relatively young males are the most frequent AAS abusers, the situation is even more alarming, since these individuals are likely to continue AAS usage throughout their lives.

One of the most worrisome psychiatric symptoms is suicidality. Suicidal ideation and suicide-related deaths have been reported to be higher in men who abuse androgens than in nonusers; a Swedish population study reported suicide-related deaths to be 22% among men abusing androgens.

Aggression. A report from the Norwegian Institute of Public Health concluded that low androgen doses influence the level of aggressiveness only slightly or not at all, but that experimental uses of the highest doses may, in some individuals, trigger mania and increased aggressiveness. In population studies, there is a clear association between the use of AAS, aggressiveness, and violence (both as perpetrator and as victim). It is not clear whether there is any causal connection.

An important review by Katinka van de Ven, of the University of New England, in Australia, states, "Although there is a growing body of research on the association between AAS and violence, results as to what the relationship is seem to be mixed." That is, "The findings show that there is a significant association between AAS use and interpersonal violence."[75] Further, "Although a meta-analytic relationship between AAS use and interpersonal violence was found, it is unclear to what extent AAS causes violent acts."

Mechanisms

Transcriptional (stimulating gene expression): This is a slow process, taking hours.

On the one hand, the classical molecular role of testosterone and other androgens in affecting cells comprises changes in the cell's gene expression, and because it is fat-soluble, testosterone can get into the nerve cell's cytoplasm and bind to an androgen receptor protein. Then, the steroid/receptor complex can get into the cell's nucleus.

Androgen receptor protein, as described by the lab of Marianne Sadar, is composed of three functional domains: the ligand-binding domain (LBD), the DNA-binding domain (DBD), and the transactivation domain (TAD).[76]

---

[75] van de Ven K, Malouff J, McVeigh J, *et al.* (2024) The association between the nonmedical use of anabolic-androgenic steroids and interpersonal violence: A meta-analysis. *J Trauma Violence Abus* **25**(2), 1484–1495.

[76] Sadar MD. (2020) Discovery of drugs that directly target the intrinsically disordered region of the androgen receptor. *Expert Opin Drug Discov* **15**(5), 551–560.

In the cell nucleus, the androgen receptor (bound by testosterone) recognizes the DNA sequence of the androgen response element, whose classical DNA sequence is GGTACAnnnTGTTCT (where "n" can be any DNA base), in various cell types. Variants of the androgen response element can also accept androgen receptor binding to activate the transcription of specific genes.

This has been a quick sketch of the classical, relatively slow mechanism of testosterone action through turning on specific genes.

Rapid, *not* transcriptional: Testosterone as an anabolic steroid can also act rapidly, independent of the genetic mechanism sketched above. For example, Yizhou Zhang and Huixian Li knew that androgens might affect synaptic function and cognition in an androgen receptor (AR)-independent manner.[77] They showed that testosterone rapidly ameliorated spatial memory deficits and neuronal damage and increased dendritic spine density and postsynaptic density protein 95. Testosterone also stimulated glutamate receptor 1 (GluA1) expression in the hippocampus in the absence of a functioning androgen receptor. Mechanistically, testosterone activated the extracellular signal-related kinase 1/2 and cyclic adenosine monophosphate response element-binding protein in the hippocampus, using mice with no functioning androgen receptors.

Another example of rapid testosterone action comes from the Kawato lab at the University of Tokyo.[78] They knew that the rapid (non-genomic) modulatory action of sex steroids (e.g.,

---

[77] Zhang Y, Chen M, Chen H, *et al.* (2024). Testosterone reduces hippocampal synaptic damage in an androgen receptor-independent manner. *J Endocrinol* **260**(2).

[78] Murakami G, Hojo Y, Kato A, *et al.* (2018) Rapid nongenomic modulation by neurosteroids of dendritic spines in the hippocampus: Androgen, oestrogen and corticosteroid. *J Neuroendocrinol* **30**(2).

testosterone, estrogens) on synapses had long been established as taking place in hippocampal neurons, established over several decades, but the essential molecular mechanisms had not been fully understood. They describe kinase-dependent signaling — enzymes that add phosphates to proteins — as mechanisms that can explain the rapid nongenomic modulation of dendritic spinogenesis in rat and mouse hippocampal slices after adding testosterone or dihydrotestosterone.

So, androgenic hormones, like testosterone, can work both by slow transcriptional mechanisms and by rapid non-transcriptional mechanisms.

Perspective

Overall, as summarized by Jorge Hallak and his team at the University of Sao Paulo, the usage of testosterone and other AAS substances aims for diminished androgenic effects while enhancing anabolic results.[79] For this reason, there are different AAS compounds and forms of usage to maximize lean body mass and blunt any side effects, such as breast development and acne.

New Challenges

As this book was going to press, the New York Times reported on "an explosion of novel lab-made chemicals that is redefining

[79] Hallak J, Teixeira TA, & de Souza GL. (2020). Effect of exogenous medications and anabolic steroids on male reproductive and sexual health, in *Male Infertility: Contemporary Clinical Approaches, Andrology, ART and Antioxidants.* Springer International Publishing, Cham, 455–468.

the illicit drug market."[80] These "ultra-potent" drugs frequently elude authorities' attempts to limit their production, and are frequently identified "only after they have shown up in the toxicology report of someone who has overdosed." What's most frightening, however, is that these drugs can be made by following reports on the internet as if they were step-by-step cookbooks. As the Times observes: "Most of these substances originate in traditional medical research, in scientific papers and patents that were published by legitimate scientists and companies and then copied and modified by illicit chemists. This is the science-to-street pipeline and it has come to dominate the illicit drug market." This pipeline runs through what is now a new synthetics frontier.

How extensive is this frontier? The Times notes that the U.N. Office on Drugs and Crime now lists 1446 new psychoactive substances, up from 643 just ten years ago. Obviously, no book can keep up with this rate of production. But we can at least comment on what this massive increase represents – the co-optation of legitimate scientific research by illegitimate operators, flooding the market with bastardized drugs whose purpose, potency, and effect may be radically altered. The identities of these drugs are masked. They are found on the street and on the dark web, all without warnings. Their market penetration is unstoppable by most conventional means, because no one wants to shut down access to scientific publication. The dilemma is terrifying when essentially anyone who understands the science can become a "cook." This new class of drugs is becoming chemistry's evil twin.

This Section of *Drugs of Abuse* demonstrates that once you understand the neurochemistry of drugs, you are better equipped to understand the new, emerging reality of drug abuse.

---

[80] https://www.nytimes.com/2026/03/31/science/drugs-psychoactive-nitazenes.html

Section 3 Three Approaches to Reducing Drug Addiction

In our studies of drugs of addiction, we encountered both pharmacological and electrophysiological techniques for blocking or avoiding aberrant drug use. We will discuss both.

Chapter I – Pharmacological Approaches

Methadone

Methadone has a dual role: It works through the brain's classical mu opioid receptor to reduce pain, but it can also be used to reduce heroin addiction by long-term occupation of the mu opioid receptor, which blocks the addictive actions of various opioids like heroin. Of course, an addict's doctor could prescribe him methadone, though there are also methadone clinics in large cities. Thus, while methadone could be abused, it is more frequently used to prevent abuse.

History. Methadone was synthesized in Germany by the Bayer Company and brought to the U.S. by U.S. health officials. The resource guide issued by the DEA states that in 1947, methadone was first used in the U.S. to reduce pain. It adds that, if misused, methadone can "lead to psychological dependence." Nonetheless, for some time, methadone has been used legally with a doctor's supervision for the purpose of reducing pain.

More than 60 years ago, a medical team at Rockefeller University led an effort to develop a pharmacotherapy for the management of heroin addiction. They hypothesized that heroin addiction is a disease of the brain with behavioral manifestations, and not merely a personality disorder, a criminal problem, or, alternatively, an antisocial personality disorder. Their pharmacologic research produced methadone. The effectiveness of methadone pharmacotherapy for combating heroin addiction is now well established.

Vulnerabilities. Genetic factors, probably involving specific small variations of multiple genes, may act in concert to enhance or reduce vulnerability to developing addictions to specific drugs, e.g., heroin or MDMA. As well, there could be early developmental changes, environmental factors (especially those that include stressful physiological and psychological impacts), and important roles for the environmental setting.

Now. Many studies have documented the ability of methadone, when used in an appropriately moderate to high dose, to prevent all narcotic abstinence signs and symptoms and reduce or prevent drug craving, thus allowing rehabilitation efforts to proceed. It is medically safe to allow someone to stay on methadone treatment in an outpatient setting, since such a patient might otherwise attempt to achieve euphoria by self-administering heroin. Outside a medical setting where methadone is administered, someone might fall back into addiction and inject heroin.

How. Methadone acts rapidly, but the duration of action is 24–36 hours (compared to 3–6 hours for heroin). That means that for up to 36 hours, the patient is protected from dangerous opioid action. Many studies concluded that it would be safe for a person to receive daily methadone treatment.

One leading researcher's understanding is that "methadone (a weak partial agonist) has a very high affinity and slow dissociation from the mu opioid receptor. As such, it can block more efficacious opioids like heroin and oxycodone from binding." It also has a much longer half-life than most opioid agonists. A major factor in the long duration of action of methadone pertains to its much slower rate of metabolism and clearance from the body than that of heroin. Because plasma levels for methadone remain elevated for long time periods, this allows for the drug to re-associate with the receptors following its dissociation, thus blocking heroin.

According to the review by Anna Ferrari at the University of Modena, in Italy, "the pharmacokinetics of methadone vary greatly from person to person."[1] So, drug concentrations will be different in different subjects. In breaking down methadone, a liver enzyme, CYP3A4, removes a methyl group (1 carbon, 3 hydrogen molecules) to produce an inactive metabolite. The activity of this enzyme also varies from person to person, such that a given dose of methadone may be too much for some patients and not enough for others.

Mechanisms. Studies from many laboratories have shown that heroin and other short-acting opiates such as morphine act primarily on the opioid system, binding at the mu-opioid receptor. It is well understood that the mu-opioid receptor is the primary site of action of several endogenous opioid peptides. It is also a major target of opioid analgesic agents and a major drug of abuse (heroin). According to the work of Eric Xu's lab in Shanghai, all the opioid peptides occupy a highly conserved "activation chamber" at the bottom of the opioid binding pit of opioid receptors,

---

[1] Ferrari A, Coccia CPR, Bertolini A, & Sternieri E. (2004) Methadone — metabolism, pharmacokinetics and interactions. *Pharmacol Res* **50**(6), 551–559.

which is engaged by an "opioid motif," e.g., the amino acids tyrosine/glycine/glycine/phenylalanine.[2] All opioid receptor ligands commonly displayed a bonding to a specific amino acid, aspartic acid, at position 149 in the mu opioid receptor's transmembrane protein 3 (TM3). Some in the field have viewed this amino acid as crucial for mu opioid receptor ligands binding.[3] This lab has also highlighted interaction with another amino acid, tyrosine, at position 150 in TM3 by means of hydrogen bonding, as critical in binding to mu opioid receptors.

It is worth noting that mutations in the gene for the mu opioid receptor are associated with opioid use disorder. This is a field of work that needs replication and extension. Science has realized the vision that heroin addiction could be addressed, at least in part, by using a rational approach to brain mechanisms, in this case by methadone blocking heroin's access to the mu opioid receptors in the brain.

Buprenorphine

About fighting heroin addiction, a comprehensive review by Sharon Walsh and her lab at the University of Kentucky built on the fact that buprenorphine is an FDA-approved medication for treatment of opioid addiction.[4] A striking example of success: During a clinical trial in France, patients who discontinued buprenorphine treatment "were ~29 times more likely to die than

---

[2] Wang Y, Zhuang Y, DiBerto JF, *et al.* (2023) Structures of the entire human opioid receptor family. *Cell* **186**(2), 413–427.e17.

[3] Coe MA, Lofwall MR, & Walsh SL. (2019) Buprenorphine pharmacology review: Update on transmucosal and long-acting formulations, *J Addict Med* **13**(2), 93–103.

[4] Id.

those who remained on buprenorphine." Here, we describe some aspects of buprenorphine use and mechanisms of its action.

Buprenorphine binds with high affinity to the same type of opioid receptor on the surface of neurons to which heroin and other full mu opioid agonists bind, but never produces the magnitude of their physiological and behavioral effects. Further, buprenorphine stays on the receptor a very long time — in the range of 20 to 40 hours, much longer than heroin or fentanyl. Such differences amongst opioids are not surprising: According to Katy Sutcliffe at the University of Bristol, different opioid molecules contact different subsets of mu opioid receptors. The bottom line? Buprenorphine efficiently blocks the most devastating and addictive actions of heroin in the brain.[5] In Sharon Walsh's words, it "reduces illicit opioid use."

Below, we highlight features of successful medical uses of buprenorphine, which include dispensing from mobile care units, combining with cognitive behavioral therapy, and using it during pregnancy.

Necessary uses of high doses

Robert Kleinman's lab in Toronto reviewed 15 studies that used high doses of buprenorphine to fight the deleterious effects of illicit fentanyl, mainly to see if such doses were safe.[6] The treatment *was* safe, and, for example, did not cause respiratory depression or fatality.

---

[5] Sutcliffe KJ, Henderson G, Kelly E, & Sessions RB. (2017) Drug binding poses relate structure with efficacy in the mu opioid receptor. *J Mol Biol* **429**(12), 1840–1851.

[6] Wong S, Fabiano N, Webber D, & Kleinman RA. (2024) High-dose buprenorphine initiation: A scoping review. *J Addict Med* **18**(4), 349–359.

Perioperative use

The Olney lab at the University of Kentucky explored the use of buprenorphine to reduce the pain of surgical operations and found that, compared to a control group, buprenorphine effectively reduced the use of more powerful "full agonists" (like heroin) at the mu opioid receptor.[7] For example, about 43% of the patients on buprenorphine avoided any use of the full agonists, whereas only 3% of the control group did. Similar results were obtained by Alexandra Vacaru and Herbert Ruckle at Loma Linda University: the buprenorphine patients used less morphine to control pain.[8]

Aurora Quaye, at Spectrum Healthcare, studied patients who had been in intensive care because of opioid addiction, following buprenorphine at the time of discharge, to see if they maintained this medication.[9] They did. In these patients, there was a significant increase in buprenorphine being prescribed 3 months post-hospital discharge by patients who had received it at the time of discharge. They did not return to illicit opioid use.

---

[7] Olney WJ, Johnson EG, Potts C, *et al.* (2023) Continuing chronic buprenorphine perioperatively is associated with reduced postoperative opioid use. *J Surg Res* **281**, 63–69.

[8] Mohammad Hajiha M, Lien D, Johnson JA, *et al.* (2023) Multimodal pain control utilizing buprenorphine for robotic-assisted laparoscopic prostatectomy: A quality improvement comparison to conventional opioid management. *Urol Pract* **10**(6), 666–670.

[9] Smith K, Wang M, Abdukalikov R, *et al.* (2022) Pain management considerations in patients with opioid use disorder requiring critical care. *J Clin Pharmacol* **62**(4), 449–462.

Combatting fentanyl

The work of Nicholas Bormann at the University of Iowa brought fentanyl into the picture.[10] Can buprenorphine successfully ease withdrawal from fentanyl by a patient with severe opioid use disorder? Yes! With high doses of buprenorphine, "the patient reported rapid improvement in withdrawal symptoms" without serious side effects. Similar success was reported by Brian Fuehrlein, at Yale, as buprenorphine "helped mitigate anhedonia and withdrawal symptoms." However, Fuehrlein also noted that "treatment dropouts are common," and that once an overdose has been reversed, "the patient remains at high risk for overdose."[11]

Mobile health units

At Brown University, Amelia Bailey and her team documented a novel approach, the provision of buprenorphine from a mobile health unit (a modified recreational vehicle). Through a scoping review of the peer-reviewed literature, she found that "delivery from the mobile unit was characterized by less stigma/judgment and greater privacy compared to fixed-site, and it was flexible and low-barrier."[12]

---

[10] Weber AN, Trebach J, Brenner MA, *et al.* (2024) Managing opioid withdrawal symptoms during the fentanyl crisis: A review. *Subst Abuse Rehabil* **15**, 59–71.
[11] Lee YK, Gold MS, Blum K, *et al.* (2024) Opioid use disorder: Current trends and potential treatments. *Front Public Health* **11**, 1274719.
[12] Bailey A, DaCunha A, Napoleon SC, *et al.* (2024) Provision of medications to treat opioid use disorder via a mobile health unit: A scoping review. *J Subst Use Addict Treat* **164**, 209431.

Cognitive behavioral therapy

Michel Perreault and his colleagues at McGill report on the value of combining buprenorphine with cognitive behavioral therapy or mindfulness to manage co-occurring chronic pain and opioid use disorder.[13] They highlight service delivery models such as integrated treatment and collaborative interdisciplinary work to tackle the multiple biopsychosocial dimensions of the co-occurring disorders. The bottom line was that the authors support "a combination of strategies to meet patient needs."

Pregnancy

Some labs in the field have tackled the problem of assessing the safety and effectiveness of buprenorphine therapy to treat opioid use disorder (OUD) during pregnancy. They were interested not only in detoxification outcomes, but also obstetrical and neonatal outcomes: "Pregnancy complications were not frequently reported. There were no reported rates of antenatal hemorrhage. Women who underwent opioid medical detoxification were found to have low rates of spontaneous abortion and intrauterine fetal demise." When detoxification was successful, neonatal pharmacological problems did not occur. Thus, careful medical application of buprenorphine to help addicted mothers during pregnancy is generally a good approach.

So, buprenorphine is really a critical tool in addressing the current crisis.

---

[13] Archambault L, Bertrand K, Martel MO, *et al.* (2024) The current state of knowledge on care for co-occurring chronic pain and opioid use disorder: A scoping review. *J Clin Nurs* **33**(8), 3056–3076.

Non-Opioid Approaches to Pain Reduction

While opioids are important to pain reduction, they entail risks, including addiction and death. Thus, it is important to consider non-opioid methods of pain reduction. Initially, these might be non-steroidal anti-inflammatory drugs (NSAIDs), such as ibuprofen, acetaminophen, and aspirin. These reduce pain and inflammation. But here we focus on an emerging approach that deals with "sodium channels."

New information on sodium channels. There is promising research about blocking certain sodium channels across the nerve cell membrane, channels that allow the flow of the positively charged ion, sodium.

Microscopic channels perforate nerve cell membranes and, in a regulated manner, allow electrically charged ions to pass through. The concentration of positively charged sodium ions is higher outside the neuron than inside, and under control by electrical fields across the membrane, positively charged sodium ions can travel through Nav channels from outside the nerve cell to inside the cell.

Sodium channels

Sodium channels consist of large proteins in the nerve cell membrane, which are closed when the electrical potential across the membrane renders the nerve cell inside 60 millivolts more negative than the extracellular fluid outside. When that electrical potential is reduced from 60 to about 55 millivolts. a segment of the protein moves toward the extracellular side of the membrane, a shift which allows positively charged sodium ions to move into the cell. This triggers the rise of the action potential, the "spike" that comprises the cell's most elementary signal.

Terminology: Sodium channels are termed "Nav" because sodium is listed in the periodic table as Na, and v is for voltage.

As reviewed by Yale professor Stephen Waxman, voltage-gated sodium channels (VGSCs) are important determinants of sensory neuron excitability with respect to pain: they are essential for the initial transduction of sensory stimuli, the electrogenesis of the action potential, and neurotransmitter release from sensory neuron terminals.[14] Nav1.1, Nav1.6, Nav1.7, Nav1.8, and Nav1.9 are all preferentially expressed by sensory neurons in adult patients. The biophysical characteristics of these channels, as well as their unique expression patterns within subtypes of sensory neurons, define their functional role in pain signaling.

Chronic pain affects one in five among the general population in the U.S. Given the poor efficacy of current analgesics, the selective expression of particular VGSCs in sensory neurons makes these attractive targets for drug discovery. The increasing availability of gene sequencing, combined with structural modeling and electrophysiological analysis of gene variants, also provides the opportunity to better target existing therapies in a personalized manner. Stephen Waxman of Yale notes that Nav1.7, Nav1.8, and Nav1.9 all contribute to the firing of peripheral pain-signaling neurons. Nav1.9 sets the baseline, from which the firing of these cells occurs. Nav1.7 amplifies small stimuli and acts to "light the fuse" for nerve impulse firing. Nav1.8 produces repetitive impulses, which cause pain. Changes in the expression of VGSCs, as well as posttranslational modifications, contribute to the sensitization of sensory neurons in chronic pain states. Furthermore, gene variants in Nav1.7, Nav1.8, and Nav1.9 have now been linked to

---

[14] Alsaloum M, Dib-Hajj SD, Page DA, *et al.* (2025) Voltage-gated sodium channels in excitable cells as drug targets. *Nat Rev Drug Discov* **24**(5), 358–378.

human genetically determined pain disorders and, more recently, to common pain disorders such as "small-fiber neuropathy."

John Wood at University College London agrees that the role of voltage-gated sodium channels like Nav1.7 and Nav1.8 in human pain sensation has been understood since the cloning of the Nav channels in the 1980s, Some channels, like Nav1.7 and Nav1.8, which have been validated through human genetics, play an important role in transmitting pain signals from peripheral sensory neurons to the central nervous system.[15]

More terminology: Among genetic mutations, so-called "gain of function" mutations yield genes that heighten the biochemical activity of the protein product. Accordingly, "loss of function" mutations produce weaker functioning proteins.

Sodium channel Nav 1.7

George Goodwin and Stephen McMahon, at Kings College London, noted that "Nav1.7 is of particular interest because individuals with Nav1.7 loss-of-function mutations are congenitally insensitive to acute and chronic pain, and there is considerable hope that phenocopying these effects with a pharmacological antagonist will produce a new class of analgesic drug."[16] Apparently, side effects present a current research problem.

A pioneer in this area, Yale professor Stephen Waxman exploited knowledge of human genetics and discovered, for example, that a gain-of-function mutation in the gene that codes Nav1.7 is associated with painful syndromes in humans. His research

---

[15] Haroun R, Gossage SJ, Iseppon F, *et al.* (2024) Novel therapies for cancer-induced bone pain. *Neurobiol Pain* **16**, 100167.

[16] Goodwin G & McMahon SB. (2021) The physiological function of different voltage-gated sodium channels in pain. *Nat Rev Neurosci* **22**(5), 263–274.

showed that certain mutations "change the biophysical properties of NaV1.7 channels leading to hyperexcitability" of certain neurons, which signal pain. His lab reported that a specific mutation, in which the amino acid methionine at position 1627 is replaced by a lysine, causes the paroxysmal extreme pain disorder due in part to rendering a particular group of pain-signaling neurons hyperexcitable.

Of great interest, David Hackos, at Genentech, genetically removed Nav1.7 in experimental mice and observed analgesia as measured by behavioral tests and by decreases in excitability of the small diameter nerve fibers, which transmit pain signals.[17]

Turning to the opposite kind of Nav1.7 manipulation, Andreas Leffler of Hanover University reported that "gain-of-function" mutations of Nav1.7 cause the pain syndromes hereditary erythromelalgia and paroxysmal extreme pain disorder.[18] In addition, several Nav1.7 mutants were shown to be associated with "small-fiber neuropathies." On the contrary, "loss-of-function" Nav1.7 mutants lead to a congenital insensitivity to pain.

Sodium channel Nav 1.8

Pharmacological approaches to Nav1.8 were called for because a loss-of-function mutation in the gene coding for Nav 1.8 reduced pain in lab animals, and increased Nav1.8's channel function due

[17] Deng L, Dourado M, Reese RM, *et al.* (2023) Nav1.7 is essential for nociceptor action potentials in the mouse in a manner independent of endogenous opioids. *Neuron* **111**(17), 2642–2659.e13.

[18] Katz D, Sindhikara D, DiMattia M, & Leffler AE. (2021) Potency-enhancing mutations of gating modifier toxins for the voltage-gated sodium channel Nav1.7 can be predicted using accurate free-energy calculations. *Toxins (Basel)* **13**(3), 193.

to mutations in human subjects correlated with painful neuropathies. Thus, an exciting development. Jim Jones and his colleagues at Vertex reported that inhibiting the function of Nav 1.8 could reduce abdominoplasty or bunionectomy pain for a period of 48 hours.[19]

Sodium channel Nav 1.9

Goodwin and McMahon note that Nav1.9's gain-of-function mutations are reported to cause congenital insensitivity to pain, so far in a very small number of individuals. But gain-of-function mutations in Nav1.9 have also been identified in individuals with clinical phenotypes associated with pain, such as painful peripheral neuropathy and familial episodic pain. Individuals who are affected complain of tingling, numbness, and pain, typically localized to the distal extremities.

Overall, Goodwin and McMahon portray pain systems as modulated by an orchestration of sodium channels, not just one channel type.

Problems remain. Some of the clinical effects of changes in sodium channel functions could be due to changes in (i) pain receptor functions, (ii) axonal electrical signaling, or (iii) neurotransmitter release, or combinations thereof. The contributions of Nav 1.7, 1.8, and 1.9 channels to pain regulation are not the same regarding these functions. Finally, some data indicate that in some cases, new drugs might have to be able to cross the blood–brain barrier for successful pain management, a formidable challenge.

---

[19] Jones J, Correll DJ, Lechner SM, *et al.* (2023) Selective inhibition of NaV1. 8 with VX-548 for acute pain. *N Eng J Med* **389**(5), 393–405.

Chapter II — Drug Addiction

Thinking about theories

Researchers commonly enquire into the motivational forces leading to the onset and maintenance of drug addiction.[20] For these researchers, both theoreticians and experimentalists, it is important to get the answers right. After all, for the year ending 31 December 2022, more than 100,000 Americans died of drug overdoses, according to the CDC. Natural and synthetic opioids, by themselves, account for more than 100,000 deaths in this country; cocaine, about 30,000 deaths. As to alcohol, the National Institute on Alcohol Abuse and Alcoholism cites more than 170,000 deaths per year due to excessive alcohol use. Regarding nicotine, more than 400,000 smoking-attributable deaths are listed in the Surgeon General's report for 2024. While death rates from all drugs have come down slightly, drug addiction is still a *major* public health problem.

Obviously, theories of drug addiction speak to issues of great public importance, but because we cannot cover all such theories here, we will focus on the clearest, most substantial, and coherent theories in neuroscience. In other words, how does neuroscience best explain how an individual becomes addicted?

In colloquial terms, one major class of theories of motivation makes use of the concept of drives (call that "push"), and another major class makes use of the concept of incentives (call that "pull"). These theories happily co-exist. Both rest on decades of careful, painstaking experimental work with human and animal subjects.

---

[20] Bandhu D, Mohan MM, Nittala NAP, *et al.* (2024) Theories of motivation: A comprehensive analysis of human behavior drivers. *Acta Psychologica* **244**, 104177.

Drives as motivational forces: Changes in bodily state, such as hunger, thirst, or sex hormones, can cause state-specific responses, such as eating, drinking, or mating, respectively. Responses must persist until the change in bodily state has been eliminated.[21]

Incentives as motivational forces: In contrast, in the absence of changes in bodily state, humans' and experimental animals' behaviors may reflect "that there are objects in the environment to which they are attracted."[22] Behavior can be motivated by the promise of rewards and modulated by those rewards' proximity and magnitude. What are the perceived values of those rewards? Tasty foods, sweetened fluids, attractive partners, and innumerable other examples render the concept of incentive motivation obvious; laboratory research supports the concept.

One leading researcher, the University of Michigan's Kent C. Berridge, working with Terry E. Robinson, has applied the literature on incentive motivation to construct the most convincing theory of addiction.[23]

Incentive salience or "wanting," as a form of motivation, depends on changes in dopaminergic neuronal systems starting in neurons of the ventral tegmental area and projected through their axons to the basal forebrain, the subcortical forebrain motor control systems called the "striatum" and to the amygdala, at least.[24]

---

[21] Cofer CN & Appley MH. (1964) *Motivation: Theory and Research*. Wiley, New York.

[22] Bolles RC. (1967) *Theory of Motivation*. Harper, New York.

[23] Robinson, TE & Berridge KC. (1993) The neural basis of drug craving: An incentive-sensitization theory of addiction. *Brain Res Rev* **18**(3), 247–291; Robinson TE & Berridge KC. (2025) The incentive-sensitization theory of addiction 30 years on. *Ann Rev Psychol* **76**(1), 29–58.

[24] Berridge KC & Robinson TE. (2016) Liking, wanting, and the incentive-sensitization theory of addiction. *Am Psychol* **71**(8), 670–679.

Signaling in these systems conveys the pleasure of certain sensory inputs (think chocolate), and increasing sensitivity in these systems results in incentives becoming irresistible. Exploding the neuronal mechanisms that underlie psychological "wanting," especially triggered by cues, makes it easy to see how an addiction could get started. Especially important are "long-lasting changes in dopamine-related motivation systems of susceptible individuals," long-lasting changes called "neural sensitization" (see below).

Experimental data are clear. For example, lesions of dopaminergic neurons abolished all motivation for food — rats would not eat and "no longer sought or consumed food rewards." The incentive-sensitization theory of addiction shows "how 'wanting' may grow over time as an individual becomes an addict, due to '*sensitization*' of brain mesolimbic systems."

Incentive salience also links naturally to the notion of anticipation. From the preceding section on Drugs of Abuse, consider, with NMDA, the anticipation of sexual arousal. For nicotine, the anticipation of the next smoke. And consider opium, leading to euphoria, not even considering the lure of the opioid fentanyl, and for cocaine, arousal coupled with feelings of reward. Anticipation is the name of the game.

Reflecting broadly on the concepts of motivation, Berridge writes that "[t]he development of addiction involves a transition from casual to compulsive patterns of drug use."[25] Over the last century or so, there have been several theoretical attempts to explain "how drug-induced alterations in psychological function might cause a transition to addiction." The most transparent among these simply emphasize the hedonic value of drug-induced

[25] Berridge KC. (2004) Motivation concepts in behavioral neuroscience. *Physiol Behav* **81**, 179–209.

pleasure and the subsequent unpleasant withdrawal symptoms. Of course, it is not difficult to imagine how an addict might be driven to additional drug use to get rid of the withdrawal symptoms (see previous section), but it is quite a challenge to enlist those to explain how addiction begins.

Other theories that Berridge considers involve learning — the view that addiction is due to aberrant learning, "especially the development of strong stimulus-response habits." But our problems with addiction have to do with primitive body signals and emotion. Perhaps abnormal patterns of activity in frontal cortical systems have something to do with addiction, but the stretch literature on those systems forces the conclusion that, while they may be related to certain cognitive aspects of addiction, the fundamental drive must come from someplace else in the brain. Berridge and Robinson thus emphasize the incentive-sensitization view, which suggests that "sensitization of a (dopaminergic) neural system that attributes incentive salience causes compulsive motivation or 'wanting' to take addictive drugs." Again, we are not here reviewing all theories of addiction; rather, we are focused on one area of research that seems most promising.

Robinson and Berridge (1993) began with the supposition that "addictive drugs share the ability to enhance mesotelencephalic dopamine neurotransmission." The enhanced operation of this system automatically signals high *incentive*, and the enhancement of activity in this system fosters *salience* to all the stimuli associated with the addictive drugs. In Berridge and Robinson's words, "Incentive salience is a psychological process that transforms the perception of stimuli, imbuing them with salience, making them attractive, 'wanted,' incentive stimuli. If this system ramps up with repeated use of addictive drugs, the addiction may become permanent."

The work of Wise and Robble is consistent with Berridge's and Robinson's thinking: "Addictive drugs are habit-forming and activate the dopamine system."[26] In one early example of experimental results, Woolverton and his team "found that rhesus monkeys would self-administer a low dose of methamphetamine only after they had received a regimen of non-contingent injections of methamphetamine."[27] In Berridge's and Robinson's terms, those low doses of methamphetamine *sensitized* dopaminergic neurons, thus to promote self-administration.

To review, from a different perspective, Berridge and Robinson's original theory (1993, 2025) argued that "repeated exposure to addictive drugs causes 'mesolimbic sensitization,' occasioned by an increase in drug-induced dopamine release; that this sensitization can last a long time even without drugs; and that the dopamine's reward value increases the salience of the incentive value of drugs, meaning that the person wants the drugs even more." Not only do the sensory cues of the drugs and the environmental triggers of repeated drug use play important roles in addiction, but even drug-related imagery can play a powerful role in sustaining drug use. Recovery is especially difficult when the former addict is surrounded by environments similar to those when (s)he became addicted.

A law of human behavior is "stimulus generalization": the tendency of a new stimulus to invoke behavioral responses just like

---

[26] Wise RA & Robble MA. (2020) Dopamine and addiction. *Ann Rev Psychol* **71**(1), 79–106.

[27] Woolverton WL, Cervo, L & Johanson CE. (1984) Effects of repeated methamphetamine administration on methamphetamine self-administration in rhesus monkeys. *Pharmacol Biochem Behav* **21**(5), 737–741.

those elicited by similar stimuli earlier.[28] This means that new environments, similar to the one that pushed the person to addiction, will foster continuing addiction. Further, recovering addicts, like all human beings, are subject to the law of Pavlovian conditioning: repeated pairing of a novel stimulus to an unconditioned stimulus will lead to conditioned responses to the novel stimulus.[29] That is, opportunities for the patient to drift back into addiction can multiply. While the bulk of research on the sensitization of mesolimbic dopamine release has been done with laboratory rodents, Berridge and Robinson cite evidence of "drug-induced behavioral sensitization in both human and non-human primates."

Recently, Jeffrey Friedman, of Rockefeller University, and Eric Nestler, of Mount Sinai have applied modern, sophisticated techniques to follow up on a large body of research showing that drugs of abuse can impact brain systems, which respond to natural rewards.[30] Their brain mapping of neuronal chemical responses to cocaine and morphine showed that neurons in a small cell group in the basal forebrain called "nucleus accumbens" are not only highly responsive to those two drugs but also manage to disrupt natural rewards: food and water consumption. There are overlapping populations of nucleus accumbens neurons responsive to drugs of abuse and natural rewards. Repeated exposures to drugs of abuse escalated this pattern of neuronal responsiveness. Studies of gene expression following exposure to cocaine or

---

[28] Pfaff D & Sherman S. (2025) *Laws of Human Behavior: Steps Toward Hard Science*. MIT Press.

[29] Id.

[30] Tan B, Browne CJ, & Nöbauer T, *et al.* (2024) Drugs of abuse hijack a mesolimbic pathway that processes homeostatic need. *Science* **384**(6693), eadk6742.

morphine allowed this team to identify a small enzyme that activates a powerful intracellular signal transduction pathway as being crucial to producing these results. Altogether, Friedman and Nestler have added detailed confirmation of the theory advanced by Berridge and Robinson, which was examined above.

Sensitization

In many papers referred to so far, the term "sensitization" is defined by behavioral measures: that a well-defined behavioral response to a drug could be obtained at lower doses than before, or that the response to a given dose would become larger. In addition to this evidence, we probed the literature for evidence of cellular and molecular phenomena that clearly could represent underlying mechanisms for neurophysiological sensitization. The earliest example we found came from the somatosensory system. In a 1965 paper in *Nature*, Lorne Mendell and Patrick Wall, working at MIT, recorded from cutaneous-responsive neurons whose axons were ascending in the dorsolateral column of the spinal cord.[31] They discovered neurons responding to repetitive combined stimulations of large-diameter and small-diameter axons with the following property: the length of the responses increased after each subsequent stimulation. So, in this phenomenon, the sensitization that produces longer responses comes simply from repetitive stimulation.

Can a sensitization phenomenon be shown for a dopaminergic system? Dopaminergic neurons that project to limbic forebrain cell groups important for addiction have indeed received some attention with respect to potential sensitization. Paulson and Robinson showed time-dependent effects of amphetamine exposure on

---

[31] Mendell LM & Wall PD. (1965) Responses of single dorsal cord cells to peripheral cutaneous unmyelinated fibres. *Nature* **206**, 97–99.

subsequent amphetamine-induced changes in behavior and dopamine release in experimental animals.[32] Likewise, in healthy humans, initial doses of amphetamine similarly led to increased dopamine release in response to subsequent amphetamine administrations.[33] Parkinson's patients with behavioral compulsions induced by their dopaminergic medications showed sensitization in response to reward-related visual cues.[34] Thus, a requirement of the incentive-sensitization theory is met by these data.

Many potential cellular mechanisms. The eight types of additional mechanisms listed below, easily gathered from recent literature, offer a vision of how ubiquitous mechanisms for neuronal sensitization (potentially applicable to Berridge's and Robinson's theory) might be. And the number of potential mechanisms certainly is not limited to eight.

Calcitonin gene-related peptide: Durham reported that the neuropeptide calcitonin gene-related peptide (CGRP) is implicated in the underlying pathology of migraine "by promoting the development of a sensitized state of primary and secondary nociceptive neurons."[35] Calcitonin is a small hormone that reduces

---

[32] Paulson PE & Robinson TE. (1995) Amphetamine-induced time-dependent sensitization of dopamine neurotransmission in the dorsal and ventral striatum: A microdialysis study in behaving rats. *Synapse* **19**(1), 56–65.

[33] Boileau I, Dagher A, Leyton M, *et al.* (2006) Modeling sensitization to stimulants in humans: An [^{11}C]raclopride/positron emission tomography study in healthy men. *Arch Gen Psychiatry* **63**(12), 1386–1395.

[34] O'Sullivan SS, Wu K, Politis M, *et al.* (2011) Cue-induced striatal dopamine release in Parkinson's disease-associated impulsive-compulsive behaviours. *Brain* **134**, 969–978.

[35] Durham PL. (2016) Diverse physiological roles of calcitonin gene-related peptide in migraine pathology: Modulation of neuronal-glial-immune cells to promote peripheral and central sensitization. *Curr Pain Headache Rep* **20**(8), 48.

blood calcium. The related CGRP, when produced in sensory systems, can be involved in the transmission of pain. Durham observed that the ability of CGRP to initiate and maintain peripheral and central sensitization is mediated by modulation of neuronal, glial, and immune cells in the trigeminal nociceptive signaling pathway. Lin and collaborators agree.[36] They wrote that within the brain, CGRP demonstrates a distinct bimodal effect, contributing to neuroprotection in some conditions while inducing neuronal sensitization and inflammation in other settings.

Nerve growth factor: Mast cells are "pharmacological bomb shells," in that they can release the chemicals histamine and heparin to great effect. They also release a lot of nerve growth factor (NGF), with the consequence of greater axonal growth in pain neurons. Of course, this leads to increased pain. Schumacher examined the role of inflammation in the nervous system in contributing to chronic pain. He observed that "inflammatory mediators, such as nerve growth factor, can lower activation thresholds of sensory neurons through modification of specific ion channels."[37]

Brain derived neurotrophic factor: Mounting evidence supports the BDNF's pro-nociceptive role, spanning from its pain-sensitizing capacity. BDNF is a protein related to NGF, which plays an obligatory role in the onset and maintenance of neuropathic pain.[38]

A potentially related function of BDNF: Microglial-derived BDNF increases synaptic activation of excitatory dorsal horn neurons and decreases that of inhibitory neurons.

---

[36] Lin K, Stiles J, Tambo W, *et al.* (2024) Bimodal functions of calcitonin gene-related peptide in the brain. *Life Sci* **359**, 123177.

[37] Schumacher MA. (2024) Peripheral neuroinflammation and pain: How acute pain becomes chronic. *Curr Neuropharmacol* **22**(1), 6–14.

[38] Smith PA. (2024) BDNF in neuropathic pain; the culprit that cannot be apprehended. *Neuroscience* **543**, 49–64.

A specific ion channel type. The "transient receptor potential cation channel subfamily V member 1" (TRPV1), also known as the capsaicin (chili pepper) receptor (burning sensations) and the Vanilloid (vanilloids, most notably capsaicin) receptor, plays a role in neuronal sensitization. The TRPV1 channel is expressed mainly in neuronal cells, more specifically, in sensory neurons responsible for the perception of noxious stimuli.[39] Adding a phosphate group to this channel's protein increases the channel's sensitization and contributes to the channel's rehabilitation after desensitization. Gao and collaborators also reviewed the evidence that sensitization of TRPV1 channels modulates sensory transmission from primary afferent nociceptors to spinal dorsal horn neurons.[40]

Multiple channels: Clinical observations of facial pain can reveal central sensitization in patients, even in the absence of visible inflammation.[41] Sensitization is characterized by a heightened responsiveness of nociceptive neurons to normal stimuli or activation by normally subthreshold stimuli, either in the peripheral or central nervous system. These heightened sensations are correlated with increased expression of multiple transient receptor potential vanilloid channels, TRPV4, TRPM3, TRPM8, TRP ankyrin 1 channels (TRPA1), Piezo2 channels, P2X3 purinergic receptors, NMDA receptors, and voltage-gated calcium channels. That is, there are more than enough channel types available to provide potential mechanisms for incentive sensitization.

---

[39] Maximiano TKE. (2024) TRPV1: Receptor structure, activation, modulation and role in neuro-immune interactions and pain. *Cell Calcium* **119**, 102870.

[40] Gao N, Li M, Wang W, *et al.* (2024) The dual role of TRPV1 in peripheral neuropathic pain: Pain switches caused by its sensitization or desensitization. *Front Mol Neurosci* **17**, 1400118.

[41] Chuinsiri N, Tiskratok W, & Jorns TP. (2024) A nociceptive-nociplastic spectrum of myofascial orofacial pain: insights from neuronal ion channel studies. *Front Cell Neurosci* **18**, 1500427.

Itch-type mechanisms: Histamine-induced itches depend on unmyelinated C-fibers, similar to pain fibers. Upon reflection, patients with intense itching display considerable somatosensory aberrations, including increased nerve sensitivity to skin stimuli as well as the perception of pain from innocuous stimuli.[42] Itch sensitization can be powered by inflammatory mediators such as bradykinin, serotonin (5-HT), and prostaglandins, leading to the activation of the NGF (see above). Histamine, as well, induces central sensitization for itch.

Epigenetics: There is no such thing as naked DNA. Instead, DNA is coated in a blanket-like fashion by basic proteins called histones. Specific amino acids in histones can be altered by chemical side groups like acetyl groups (enhance access to DNA) or methyl groups (usually reduce access to DNA). These histone modifications comprise "epigenetics" (etymology, "beyond" genetics). It now appears that such histone modifications can be relevant to sensitization.

Recently, in the work of Zhang and collaborators, the elevated activity of histone deacetylase (HDAC) has emerged as a key mechanism contributing to the development and maintenance of neuropathic pain.[43] HDACs, widely distributed in sensory neurons of the spinal cord, regulate gene expression by deacetylation of histone proteins, resulting in increased neuronal excitability and neuroinflammation, thus promoting peripheral and central sensitization. Importantly, pharmacological manipulation of aberrant

---

[42] Yosipovitch G, Kim B, Luger T, *et al.* (2024) Similarities and differences in peripheral itch and pain pathways in atopic dermatitis. *J Allergy Clin Immunol* **153**(4), 904–912.

[43] Zhang W, Jiao B, Yu S, *et al.* (2024) Histone deacetylase as emerging pharmacological therapeutic target for neuropathic pain: From epigenetic to selective drugs. *CNS Neurosci Thera* **30**(5), e14745.

acetylation using HDAC-targeted inhibitors (HDACi) has shown promising pain-relieving properties in various preclinical models of neuropathic pain. Zhang and collaborators feel that abnormally elevated levels of certain HDACs promote neuronal excitability and neuroinflammation by epigenetically modulating pivotal gene expression in neuronal and immune cells, thus contributing to central sensitization in the progression of neuropathic pain. Also, recent studies from the lab of Yize Li have identified the involvement of euchromatic histone-lysine N-methyltransferase 2 in neuropathic pain associated with the transcriptional silencing of many potassium ion channel genes.[44] This would allow higher frequencies of neuronal firing, and, in that sense, sensitization. Are there epigenetic changes in mesencephalic dopaminergic neurons that could contribute to incentive sensitization?

Morphological changes in sensitization: Inevitably, some features of neuronal sensitization will involve morphological features. Oliva and collaborators hold that the elucidation of synaptic density changes provides valuable insights into the underlying brain mechanisms of behavioral sensitization and drug self-administration in rodents.[45] Notably, hippocampal spine density increased after amphetamine; amphetamine, cocaine, and nicotine all increased spine density in the nucleus accumbens. Whether these morphological changes represent the causes, effects, or both, of behavioral sensitization remains to be discovered.

---

[44] Zhang Q, Ding R, Li Y,*et al.* (2024) Euchromatin histone-lysine N-methyltransferase 2 regulates the expression of potassium-sodium-activated channel subfamily T member 1 in primary sensory neurons and contributes to remifentanil-induced pain sensitivity. *Brain Res Bull* **212**(Pt 3), 110966.

[45] Oliva HNP, Prudente TP, Nunes EJ, *et al.* (2024) Substance use and spine density: A systematic review and meta-analysis of preclinical studies. *Mol Psychiatry* **29**(9), 2873–2885.

Outlook

In sum, we need a coherent theory for neuroscientists to move forward in a rational manner, toward understanding how drugs of abuse grab control of human behavior. Incentive-sensitization theory is intellectually coherent and has substantial empirical support. Therefore, its predictions for the results of sophisticated behavioral studies in the lab, followed by clinical applications, provide the best chance of beating drug addiction.

Section 4 For the Future: Paths Toward Recovery?

Prior sections of this book examined the origins of some drugs of abuse, as well as brain mechanisms involved in the operation of many such drugs. This section looks at possible brain-based interventions to curb drug abuse. Such reverse engineering could be fascinating: While we know that brain mechanisms play a part in developing addictive behaviors, it may now be that they can lead the way out. Of course, these approaches may seem speculative, even futuristic. Moreover, as drug abuse evolves, with new drugs coming on the market, there is an increased willingness to depart from conventional treatments. There is a "we'll-try-anything" attitude reflecting a relative lack of success so far.

We highlight these potentially speculative approaches because their methodologies radically and deliberately depart from older approaches, e.g., 12-Step programs, which are unable to curtail drug abuse across a wide spectrum of users. These newer approaches, some still untested, help to understand *why* the older approaches may not be adequate. They often start from fundamentally different premises about the nature of addiction and the personality of the addict. Finally, we will discuss the older approaches by way of comparison to the newer, still-emerging ideas, so that readers can make their own judgments concerning what types of adaptations may be useful in drug treatment modalities.

We begin with some new reflections from a "futurologist," lawyer/philosopher Nita Farahany. The next few paragraphs closely follow Farahany's book. Then, we describe various approaches to combating addiction.

In *The Battle for Your Brain* (2023), Nita Farahany writes (p. 3): "Globally, the market for neurotechnology is growing at a compound annual rate of 12 percent and is expected to reach 21 billion [dollars] by 2026."[1] What is "neurotechnology" in context with drug abuse? In effect, it is a type of popular, commercially available tech that allows people to monitor their brain function and, hence, follow the effect of drugs — and drug withdrawal — in real time. In private, an individual can track their own electroencephalographs (EEGs) and even see reports of the blood flow in the brain. By analogy, if diabetics track their blood sugar level throughout the day, the same well-accepted principle could be applied to addiction ("Are the electric pulses in my brain anomalous?" "Is the blood flow spiking?"). Likewise, many people track various vital functions when they exercise (e.g., through Apple watches). Farahany would only take the technology a step further, albeit in another direction. She makes this approach seem almost inevitable (p.11): "Self-tracking is far more than a fad. It is a new way of living and thinking about ourselves."

To the extent that people are more comfortable taking charge of their own rehab (rather than having the government or an institution take charge), "self-tracking" would be huge. It would allow drug abusers to experience agency, whereas most of the time they feel — rightly or wrongly — that they are subject to control by someone with an "agenda." The theory is that if they can watch what is happening in their brains 24/7, rather than having someone

---

[1] Farahany NA. (2023) *The Battle for Your Brain: Defending the Right to Think Feely in the Age of Neurotechnology*. St. Martin's Press, London.

tell them during a weekly appointment, they will be incentivized to help bring their brain activity into conformity with some sort of norm. They will be less resentful of and resistant toward treatment.

Such self-determination, "understood to be free from governmental interference when making decisions that only affect oneself," (136) has philosophical roots in Immanuel Kant and John Stuart Mill (18th and 19th centuries, respectively). Individuals are free to make choices so long as they do not harm the interests of others. In theory, any option that hurts no one else — even apart from neurotechnology — would be available to an addict seeking to quit.

Farahany favors self-directed approaches to recovery from addiction, noting that "When society interferes with purely personal conduct, it invariably does so wrongly and in the wrong place." (144) This is an overstatement. Nonetheless, she has a point. Her rationale is grounded in "Theory of Mind," the ability to understand the thoughts and feelings of other people. In effect, Farahany is attempting to understand the mind of an addict, not an entirely presumptuous effort in that, for a time, she was one. She says that "equipped with Theory of Mind we try to influence and persuade people around us." Theory of Mind refers to our ability to intuit the intentions and feelings of other humans. We could influence and persuade an addict to take charge of their addiction, rather than trying to influence and persuade the addict by *our* taking charge.

We know that neurons involved in "theory of mind behavior" include those in the prefrontal cortex (PFC) and those at the juncture of the temporal and parietal lobes of the brain. Because it is well understood (at least from a neuroscience perspective), "Theory of Mind" lends practical support to Farahany's idea that we encourage addicts to make useful positive changes.

But how far to take Farahany? Should encouragement tip into manipulation ("Oh, it's for their own good!")? Some scholars describe patient manipulation as "interfering with their mental integrity," namely, "the individual's mastery of his mental states and his brain data." So, they would prohibit unconsented-to interferences. The trick is to obtain a patient's consent to self-tracking, which they could hardly do without providing consent, unless any neurotechnology they used were to be read remotely, without their knowledge. That seems highly unlikely and, indeed, much more futuristic than anything Farahany proposes; her approach is based on allowing an addict to experience a newfound agency in the conduct of their treatment.

What about other sorts of influence on curbing addictive behavior? Farahany observes that "Advertisers have gotten much better at identifying and targeting our baked-in desires. People are unaware of the powerful influences brought to bear on their choices and behavior." Advertising is not in itself coercive. It may weaken our will, e.g., to consume drugs, but we still retain the agency to resist. (p. 163) The question is whether disabling our will — at least over the long run — is tantamount to coercion (and is that so bad in the context of drugs? Is it worse if the subject doesn't realize the underlying intent of the ads?). As to behavior-altering ads, some advertisers talk about subliminal "priming" of a subject's thoughts or feelings. The concept refers to the potential ability of a prior sensory stimulus, which is below the subject's threshold for detection (subliminal), to influence the subject's subsequent response to another, easily detected stimulus. The "priming" would appeal to our common sense, offering a simple and potentially attractive (if not entirely ingenuous) idea. But the essence of the scientific endeavor depends on the production and reports of scientific results, which can be repeated by other scientists in other laboratories. "Subliminal priming" did not pass that test; studies reporting it were not routinely replicated by work in other laboratories. So, this type of priming does not appear to be an effective weapon and would not interfere with efforts to afford drug abusers greater agency in curtailing their abuse.

The question is how much agency. Because institutions could still help initiate addicts into a self-help regime, it is unlikely that Farahany would disallow their role entirely. But she *would* shift the balance between individual and institutional actors in dealing with drug abuse. Here are some of her proposals in that regard, as well as others in that spirit:

Electrical stimulation of the human brain. The somewhat vague concept of "neurofeedback" is invoked in claims that the everyday brain-trainer can buy an EEG device that, in some way, will reinforce the learning process (p. 113). Elon Musk's company, Neurolink, wants to implant electrodes in the brain to use brain/computer linkages to help patients with movement disorders. In fact, this kind of technological attempt has been pursued for years in a variety of labs. In the future, it may be possible for this type of brain-training, coupled with powerful machine learning technology, to empower self-control, including training oneself to recover from addiction.

Electrical stimulation of the human brain has long been used, for example, to help Parkinson's Disease patients (Mahlon DeLong at Emory), for speech problems (Edward Chang at UCSF), and for problems of disordered consciousness (Nicholas Schiff, at Cornell Medical).

Farahany believes that we are "at a stalemate at best" (p. 140) in battling the opioid epidemic. Taking a radical approach, Chinese medical scientists tried damaging the reward-associated nucleus accumbens of 11 patients (p. 141). But that proved so controversial that the trial was halted. Deep brain stimulation (DBS) is likely to offer better options for battling addiction, especially now because, using up-to-date techniques, we can limit the neurons affected by using (a) low currents with tiny electrodes, and (b) virological techniques to target specific neuron types.

Could the concept of "neuromarketing" (p. 148) help? Professor Morton Cerf, Northwestern University, is one of many proponents of "neuromarketing," which usually means using ultrasensitive physiological measures to track subjects' internal reactions to stimuli of commercial importance. Subjects in such surveys may not be aware of what these internal reactions are, or their significance to the companies whose products are being tested. Methods for measuring reactions could include EEG, electrocardiological (ECG) signals from the heart, emotion-related pupil responses, functional magnetic resonance imaging (fMRI), and sweating on the skin. Some of these measures could reflect unconscious emotional reactions to the companies' products or advertising.

Bazzani and collaborators review that companies have benefited from tracking these emotional reactions, and particularly emphasize the successful use of EEG.[2] Nevertheless, the startling particularity of certain findings (e.g., "prefrontal asymmetry in the gamma oscillation bands") makes the skeptical neuroscientist wonder which are (a) the reliable results of commercial value or (b) some combination of questionable technique and wishful thinking.

Hakim and Levy celebrate the ability of sensitive physiological measurements to transcend "limitations of traditional marketing techniques, such as questionnaires, focus groups, and interviews,"

---

[2] Bazzani A, Ravaioli S, Trieste L, *et al.* (2020) Is EEG suitable for marketing research? A systematic review. *Front Neurosci* **14**, 594566.

and emphasize the use of EEGs.[3] The main problem here will be to avoid overinterpretation of minor EEG changes, particularly those that favor a company's preferences. Stasi and collaborators commend "Consumer Neuroscience as a new burgeoning field comprising academic research at the intersection of neuroscience, psychology, economics, decision theory, and marketing," and apply themselves to food-related decision-making processes.[4] So, for example, they report that fMRI studies have been useful to understand which brain areas are enrolled in the decision-making process, so that they can be proficiently applied for future research.

The desideratum will be the use of these internal neurological and other physiological signals, of which the potential consumer is unaware, to guide companies' strategies as they choose to produce and market certain foods. Of course, for our current project, we want to see these techniques applied to enable recovery from drug addiction.

Chemical assistance in reducing dependence on drugs

"Making cognitive enhancers available to individuals" (Farahany, p. 129) gives those individuals opportunities to use or forego. The use of cognitive enhancers can be regulated to (a) make sure they are safe and effective, and (b) preserve society's interests.

On the other hand, a traumatized woman sought help from a psychiatrist at Harvard Medical School who studies post-traumatic

---

[3] Hakim A & Levy DJ. (2019) A gateway to consumers' minds: Achievements, caveats, and prospects of electroencephalography-based prediction in neuromarketing. *Wiley Interdiscip Rev Cogn Sci* **10**(2), e1485.

[4] Stasi A, Songa G, Mauri M, *et al.* (2018) Neuromarketing empirical approaches and food choice: A systematic review. *Food Res Int* **108**, 650–664.

stress disorder (Farahany, p. 130). The psychiatrist was uncertain how to handle her case, but to possibly prevent a full-fledged return to the horror she had witnessed, he suggested that she try an experimental use of propranolol (a blocker of excitatory neurochemicals like adrenaline).

Farahany traces (p. 112) increases in the rate at which "healthy people take brain-enhancing drugs," e.g., Adderall and Ritalin, for attention deficit hyperactivity disorder. There are circumstances where psychoactive drugs could help with recovery from addiction. Medicinal viral microinjections into the brain will be coming along soon, with the intention of altering the firing rates of specific types of neurons in the service of relieving drug cravings.

Overall, Dr. Ahmed Shaheed (p. 165) agrees that all kinds of influence and persuasion are acceptable, but at some point, "an influence crosses the line from permissible persuasion to impermissible manipulation." Consider: (a) Has the addict consented to the practice, (b) Would a reasonable person be aware of it, (c) Is there a power imbalance between influence and addict? and (d) Is there actual harm to the addict? An answer pattern of "Yes, Yes, No, No" would be ideal for moving ahead with the helpful attempt.

Drug Addiction Treatments in Practice

The Addicted Brain (2023) by neuroscientist Michael J. Kuhar lists seven websites that can help with withdrawal (p. 190) and several principles for adequate treatment, including ready availability 24/7, a qualified caregiver, the necessity to stay in treatment, and continual assessment of progress and readiness of treatment modifications to meet the patient's changing needs. Kuhar recommends medicines, including, for nicotine, bupropion (an antidepressant), and varenicline (works through the brain's nicotinic acetylcholine receptor); for alcohol, disulfiram (Antabuse); and for opioids, methadone or buprenorphine. Different individuals need different approaches.[5] One size does not fit all.

If untreated, opioid use disorder (OUD) is associated with significant morbidity and mortality. However, addicts can rarely manage their recovery without assistance. Some effective approaches to opioid addiction are covered by Jessica Taylor and Jeffrey Samet (2022): Buprenorphine and methadone (see above) reduce fatal and nonfatal opioid overdose and infectious complications of opioid use and are the first-line treatment options.

Another compound, Naltrexone, is an opioid antagonist that, however, does not address withdrawal symptoms. Patients must abstain from opioids for 7 to 10 days before initiation, depending on the half-life of the opioids used. Thus, patients in opioid withdrawal awaiting naltrexone treatment usually require management of withdrawal symptoms with other agents during this washout period.

A retrospective comparative effectiveness study compared the effect of various treatments to no treatment. Compared with no treatment, only buprenorphine and methadone were associated with decreased opioid overdose and opioid-related acute care at both 3 and 12 months. Non-intensive behavioral health was associated with a decrease in opioid-related acute care, a marginal gain at months 3 and 12, and a reduction in opioid overdose at month 12 but not month 3.

---

[5] Kuhar MJ. (2023) *The Addicted Brain*. Pearson Education, Inc

James Bell and John Strang concur that methadone (a full opioid agonist), buprenorphine (a partial agonist), and naltrexone (an opioid antagonist) are effective for OUD.[6] Methadone and buprenorphine act by suppressing opioid withdrawal symptoms and attenuating the effects of other opioids. Naltrexone blocks the effects of opioid agonists. Another medication mode of minimizing the risk of overdose is take-home naloxone, the opioid antagonist used to reverse opioid overdose; take-home naloxone programs aim to prevent fatal overdose.

Bell and Strang further agree that current standards of care for medically supervised withdrawal include treatment with μ-opioid receptor agonists (e.g., methadone), partial agonists (e.g., buprenorphine), and $\alpha 2$-adrenergic receptor agonists (e.g., clonidine and lofexidine). Newer agents likewise exploit these pharmacological mechanisms, including tramadol (μ-opioid receptor agonism) and tizanidine ($\alpha 2$ agonism). Areas for future research include managing withdrawal in the context of stabilizing patients with OUD to *extended-release naltrexone*, transitioning patients with OUD from methadone to buprenorphine, and *tapering opioids* in patients with chronic, non-cancer pain.

Another new approach is to use clonidine, which treats opioid withdrawal symptoms through its anti-adrenergic actions, specifically targeting noradrenergic hyperactivity in locus coeruleus neurons that cause opioid withdrawal symptoms. Alternatively, extended-release naltrexone is a viable treatment for OUD, and monthly injections could be especially useful for patients who struggle with adherence and are prone to agonist diversion or misuse.

---

[6] Bell J & Strang J. (2020) Medication treatment of opioid use disorder. *Biol Psychiatry* **87**(1), 82–88.

Glucagon-like peptides (GLPs)

Martinelli and collaborators (2024) presented evidence suggesting that GLP-1 receptor agonists (GLP-1RA) have a potential use in addiction treatment. 1218 studies were analyzed. The therapeutic effectiveness of GLP-1RA on SUD (substance use disorders) was assessed in 5 of the studies, with 3 demonstrating a significant decrease in SUD (alcohol and nicotine). GLP-1RA's impact on body weight, BMI, and HbA1c was reported in three studies. These revealed a notable reduction in these parameters among the GLP-1RA-treated group. They concluded that GLP-1RA in SUD is a possible new option for therapy in addiction medicine. Herman and Schmidt agreed: glucagon-like peptide-1 receptor (GLP-1R) agonists attenuate voluntary nicotine taking and seeking and prevent withdrawal-induced hyperphagia and body weight gain.[7] "Emerging evidence also suggests that GLP-1R agonists improve cognitive deficits, as well as depressive- and anxiety-like behaviors, which contribute to smoking relapse during withdrawal." In sum, the current literature supports GLP-1R-based approaches to treating nicotine addiction.

Electrical or magnetic stimulation

Animal brains. Wang and collaborators also recognized that new therapies were needed to combat drug addiction, and that DBS might be an effective treatment.[8] The past 15 years saw numerous

---

[7] Herman RJ & Schmidt HD. (2024) Targeting GLP-1 receptors to reduce nicotine use disorder: Preclinical and clinical evidence. *Physiol Behav* **281**, 114565.

[8] Wang TR, Moosa S, Dallapiazza RF, *et al.* (2018) Deep brain stimulation for the treatment of drug addiction. *Neurosurg Focus* **45**(2), E11.

animal DBS studies on the addiction to various drugs of abuse, with most reporting decreases in drug-seeking behavior with stimulation. The most common target for stimulation has been the nucleus accumbens, a key structure in the mesolimbic reward pathway. The prefrontal cortex, as well as other targets involved in drug addiction, such as the lateral habenula, hypothalamus, insula, and subthalamic nucleus, have also been stimulated in animals, with encouraging results. Although animal studies have largely shown promising results, current DBS studies for drug addiction primarily use stimulation during active drug use. More data is needed on the effect of DBS during withdrawal in preventing future relapse.

Human brains. Mehta and collaborators felt that while pharmacological and behavioral treatments are available for substance use disorders, they are not always effective or well-tolerated.[9] Neuromodulation methods, including repetitive transcranial magnetic stimulation, transcranial direct current stimulation, and DBS, may address SUDs by targeting neural circuitry involved in the maintenance of addictive behaviors. They evaluated the efficacy of neuromodulation to improve human behavioral outcomes in SUDs. A total of 94 studies was reviewed. "Results were most encouraging when multiple stimulation sessions were applied, and the left dorsolateral prefrontal cortex (DLPFC) was targeted. Transcranial direct current stimulation also produced medium effect sizes for drug use and craving, though they were highly variable and less robust than transcranial magnetic stimulation; right anodal (positive charged) DLPFC stimulation appeared to be most efficacious."

---

[9] Mehta DD, Praecht A, Ward HB, *et al.* (2024) A systematic review and meta-analysis of neuromodulation therapies for substance use disorders. *Neuropsychopharmacology*, **49**(4), 649–680.

Soleimani and collaborators reviewed 205 studies that used brain stimulation to reduce addiction. Whereas most previous clinical trials targeted the dorsolateral prefrontal cortex, accumulating data highlight the frontopolar cortex as a promising therapeutic target for transcranial brain stimulation in SUDs.[10] Treatments were most successful when they were accompanied by a trained recovery coach to help the addicted patient.

Fatemizadeh and collaborators note that the anterior cingulate cortex has been implicated in various types of SUDs, including nicotine, heroin, and alcohol use disorders, and thus aimed to investigate the effects of DBS in the anterior cingulate cortex as a potential therapeutic approach for morphine use disorder.[11] Findings indicate that high-frequency (130 Hz) DBS at different amperages, 150 μA and 200 μA in the anterior cingulate cortex during the acquisition phase of morphine conditioned place preference (CPP, a quantitative measure of the animal's addiction), inhibited the rewarding properties of morphine. Furthermore, DBS at these intensities during the reduction in tendency toward addiction facilitated the loss and opposed the reinstatement of morphine addiction triggered by experimental drug priming. In conclusion, these data indicated an intensity-dependent effect of anterior cingulate cortex DBS on the acquisition, extinction, and reinstatement of morphine-induced CPP in rats. These findings suggest that anterior cingulate cortex DBS could be a potential intervention for the treatment of morphine use disorder.

---

[10] Soleimani G, Joutsa J, Moussawi K, *et al.* (2024) Converging evidence for frontopolar cortex as a target for neuromodulation in addiction treatment. *Am J Psychiatry* **181**(2), 100–114.

[11] Fatemizadeh M, *et al.* (2025) Deep brain stimulation of the anterior cingulate cortex reduces opioid addiction in preclinical studies. *Sci Rep* **15**, 2065.

Treiber and collaborators reported that transcranial magnetic stimulation reduced alcohol craving over sham stimulation immediately post-treatment.[12] Concerning a maintenance effect, a meta-analysis revealed a medium effect for active transcranial magnetic stimulation in the reduction of alcohol craving at a 3-month follow-up. A subgroup analysis revealed that transcranial magnetic stimulation targeting the medial PFC may be more effective than stimulating the right dorsolateral PFC or left dorsolateral PFC immediately after treatment. The authors concluded that a minimum of 10 sessions of transcranial magnetic stimulation reduced alcohol craving immediately after treatment; this effect seems to be sustained over a 3-month period.

Thus, DBS in humans can be effective in reducing drug addiction, but, so far, studies have not zeroed in on one "magic" location for stimulation.

Quitting a stimulant drug. Li and Shoptaw estimated that a majority of people who use psychostimulants, particularly methamphetamine and cocaine, experience withdrawal upon abstinence from sustained use.[13] What is the evidence regarding biomedical and behavioral treatments for psychostimulant withdrawal symptoms? Potential efficacy for methamphetamine withdrawal is noted for a few medications. In addition to naltrexone and bupropion (mentioned above), mirtazapine, an antidepressant, showed promise. Also, repetitive transcranial magnetic stimulation during the acute (first week), early protracted (weeks 2–4),

---

[12] Treiber M, Tsapakis EM, & Fountoulakis K. (2025) Repetitive transcranial magnetic stimulation for alcohol craving in alcohol use disorders: A meta-analysis. *J Addict Med* **19**(2), 195–201.

[13] Li MJ & Shoptaw SJ. (2023) Clinical management of psychostimulant withdrawal: Review of the evidence. *Addiction* **118**(4), 750–762.

and late protracted (>4 weeks) withdrawal phases aided stimulant drug withdrawal.

Kundal and collaborators tried a surprising approach — "Rhemercise," a novel mindfulness technique, was used to prevent relapse in OUD.[14] It is a quantifiable and intentional slow-breathing technique that could increase subjective well-being, which helps to prevent relapse in OUD by reducing craving, negative affect, and visceral reactivity. Various domains of the Subjective Well-Being Inventory (general well-being-positive effect, confidence in coping, inadequate mental mastery) improved significantly among OUD patients who received rhemercise treatment compared to treatment as usual. Thus, according to this study, "Rhemercise" promoted general well-being and positive affect and decreased the opioid withdrawal symptoms, thereby potentially reducing the overall risk for relapse.

Reducing relapse

Patel and Kosten focused on methods to reduce relapse and optimize treatment strategies. That is, once a patient completes withdrawal and establishes sobriety regarding illicit opioids, the maintenance stage of treatment includes the corresponding danger of relapse.[15] There are several different pharmacological treatment options, including a full mu-opioid agonist (methadone), a partial mu-opioid agonist (buprenorphine), and a mu-opioid antagonist

---

[14] Kundal D, Raj R, Garg R, *et al.* (2022) Therapeutic efficacy of rhemercise: A novel mindfulness technique in patients with opioid use disorder. *Prim Care Companion CNS Disord* **24**(1), 21m03064.

[15] Patel B & Kosten TR. (2019) Keeping up with clinical advances: Opioid use disorder. *CNS Spectr* **24**(S1), 14–24.

(naltrexone). Psychosocial interventions are also beneficial, including group and individual counseling, sober living centers, partial hospitalization programs, and residential long-term treatment.

Further help in preventing relapse comes from the development of extended-release opioid blocker naltrexone.[16] The emergence of extended-release naltrexone raises the opportunity to explore the role of endorphin blockade on hedonic response during long-term alcohol dependence treatment. A hedonic survey — a survey of subjects' emotions — was administered to 74 alcohol-dependent patients treated for an average of 3.5 years, with nearly continuous month-long intramuscular XR-NTX. The paper-and-pencil, one-time survey asked patients about the degree of pleasure they experienced in the past 90 days with drinking alcohol, sex, exercise, and other daily activities. The data revealed lower pleasure ratings for alcohol than for sex, exercise, and 10 other common activities. Mean responses to drinking alcohol and gambling were significantly lower than to listening to music, sex, reading, being with friends, eating good food, eating spicy food, and playing video/card games. This effect was independent of XR-NTX dose or duration. Although this exploratory study lacked baseline data, a comparison group, or a control for the impact of patient discontinuation, the data indicate the feasibility of examining long-term hedonic response in recovery. The differential hedonic ratings suggest that in patients who persist with long-term continuous therapy, XR-NTX may selectively inhibit the pleasure associated with drinking alcohol, compared to a variety of other activities.

Once a patient is in the maintenance stage of treatment, methadone maintenance or office-based buprenorphine therapy

---

[16] Coviello DM, Cornish JW, Lynch KG, *et al.* (2010) A randomized trial of oral naltrexone for treating opioid-dependent offenders. *Am J Addict* **19**(5), 422–432.

can help manage opioid cravings and prevent acute and reduce protracted withdrawal symptoms. Risk factors for relapse include psychosocial factors that cannot be addressed by psychopharmacology alone, such as unstable housing and lack of employment. Other risk factors include current cocaine or alcohol use and social factors such as living with a heroin user. The importance of psychosocial interventions is to address the psychological and social stressors patients are facing.

Continuing problems with withdrawal

David and collaborators asked patients to identify continuing barriers to a successful withdrawal from drugs. They cited: (1) a lack of continuity of care, (2) a limited number of detox and residential treatment program beds, (3) unstable housing, and (4) a lack of options when choosing a treatment pathway.[17] Solutions proposed by participants included: (1) increasing the low-barrier access to community opioid use, (2) adding case managers at the detox center to establish a continuity of care after discharge, (3) increased assistance with housing, and (4) encouraging patient participation in treatment decisions. Overall, patients identified the lack of continuity of care, especially care coordination, as a major barrier to substance use treatment. Increasing treatment utilization, including medications for opioid use disorder, necessitates a multimodal approach to the continuity of care, low-barrier access to getting medicine, and support to address unstable housing. Patients want care that incorporates options and respect for individualized preferences and needs.

---

[17] David AR, Sian CR, Gebel CM, *et al.* (2022) Barriers to accessing treatment for substance use after inpatient managed withdrawal (detox): A qualitative study. *J Subst Abuse Treat* **142**, 108870.

How to deal with these continuing problems? Addiction expert Charles P. O'Brien, professor of psychiatry at the University of Pennsylvania, argues that "both pharmacotherapy and behavioral treatments are required to relieve the symptoms of addictive disorders." Further, he states that treatments must be long-term, measured in months and years, and that they must be specific to the individual (p. 277). In light of his experience and convincing arguments, how do we view the efforts of three of the best-known addiction clinics in the U.S.?

Special case: getting off methamphetamine. It can be extremely difficult for methamphetamine users to stop using meth, even to the point where patients die rather than stop. Recently, a behavioral approach called "contingency management" has been instituted in some services with a simple arrangement: take a day off meth and get some cash. Newspaper-level reporting (*The New York Times*) says that such contingency management works. Lake and collaborators write that "findings highlight the opportunity for behavioral treatment programs to tailor program structures to individual-specific characteristics."[18]

Three Clinics with Divergent Approaches to Fighting Addiction

Medically supervised organizations have, over the years, acquired substantial knowledge regarding the treatment of addicts. Nonetheless, their self-described treatment modalities vary widely,

[18] Lake MT, Krishnamurti T, Murtaugh KL, *et al.* (2023) Decision-making tendencies and voucher spending independently support abstinence within contingency management for methamphetamine use disorder. *Exp Clin Psychopharmacol* **31**(2), 324–329.

e.g., from the old-fashioned 12-step approach (Minnesota Model) to a more recent harm reduction approach (Passages).

The **Minnesota Model** of caring for the addict claims that "there is no 'cure' just an ability to stop the illness from being active, 'one day at a time.' In other words, the alcoholic's and addict's problems are long term, they don't just go away." Assumptions behind the Minnesota Model (stated in terms of alcoholism) are that: "Alcoholism exists; it is an illness and those with the illness have no control over their drinking. It is a no-fault illness which affects those suffering physically, mentally, and spiritually." This model of care also applies to drug addiction.

The model can be summed up as: Medical treatment, seeking "total abstinence and complete surrender — and an admission that alcoholics cannot manage life if they use alcohol in any form." It uses the12-step treatment program from Alcoholics Anonymous, largely reliant on religion:

Step 1: We admitted we were powerless over alcohol — that our lives had become unmanageable.

Step 2: Came to believe that a Power greater than ourselves could restore us to sanity.

Step 3: Made a decision to turn our will and our lives over to the care of God as we understood .him

Step 4: Made a searching and fearless moral inventory of ourselves.

Step 5: Admitted to God, to ourselves, and to another human being the exact nature of our wrongs.

Step 6: We were entirely ready to have God remove all these defects of our character.

Step 7: Humbly asked Him to remove our shortcomings.

Step 8: Made a list of persons we had harmed and became willing to make amends to them all.

Step 9: Made direct amends to such people wherever possible, except when to do so would injure them or others.

Step 10: Continued to take personal inventory and, when we were wrong, promptly admitted it.

Step 11: Sought through prayer and meditation to improve our conscious contact with God, as we understood Him, praying only for the knowledge of His will for us and the power to carry that out.

Step 12: Having had a spiritual awakening as a result of these Steps, we tried to carry this message to alcoholics, and to practice these principles in all our affairs.

The 12 steps are purported to work because they involve admitting to a problem and seeking to correct it; seeking help from others with a similar problem, who can therefore empathize; calling on one's spirituality (assuming it exists) and using it to one's advantage. The Model rigidly focuses on human wrongdoing — in a Judeo-Christian, fallen sense — and draws from that the necessity for total abstinence, i.e., reversing the wrong. It does not accommodate non-believers, and the reference to a male God (see Step 3) may be offensive to women and even people along the LGBTQ spectrum.[19] It is not based on harm reduction (see following section) and does not accept notions of human agency to craft one's mode of treatment (apart from total abstention). It is essentially a one-size-fits-all approach. Based on hard statistics, however, it has been

[19] Greene D. (2021) Revisiting 12-step approaches: An evidence-based perspective, in *Addictions — Diagnosis and Treatment*.

criticized as insufficiently capable of keeping most people involved and, therefore, as unable to bring about long-term recovery.[20]

The **Geisinger Marworth Treatment Center**, in Waverly, Pennsylvania, specializes in addiction treatment for uniformed professionals. Specialists at Geisinger recognize that "for those who work in uniform, the fast-paced, often stressful environment can be challenging, which can cause people to turn to alcohol or drugs and develop an addiction." Tip-offs that a public servant might be addicted could include, for example, frequent absences, decline in work performance, changes in appearance, or hygiene. Of course, it is easy to imagine potential contributing causes of addiction, including, in Geisinger's words, exposure to trauma, PSTD, and risks of physical danger, with all of these potentially straining family dynamics. Its treatments include medications, such as methadone, buprenorphine, and naltrexone, intensive group therapy with other uniformed professionals, grief counseling, stress management training, and recurrent use-prevention groups designed especially for uniformed professionals.

Marworth also offers additional services to support those recovering from alcohol or drug addiction as they seek to maintain sobriety. For relapse prevention, it now offers an outpatient Stage-Two Recovery Group, which "is ideal for patients who have demonstrated stabilization in their individual recovery process and express an interest in improving their relationships with themselves and others through further group therapy experiences."

At the **Betty Ford Clinic in Malibu, CA, now called Passages Malibu**, the operators seek to follow what they consider a holistic addiction treatment philosophy. Like Marworth, they do

---

[20] Dodes L & Dodes Z. (2015) *The Sober Truth: Debunking the Bad Science Behind 12-Step Programs and the Rehab Industry*. Beacon Press.

not follow the 12-step program: "At Passages Malibu, we focus on healing the underlying conditions that are causing you to use drugs and alcohol. We do this by utilizing a highly individualized treatment program with therapists who are experienced in healing the underlying causes of addiction. They do not use the 12 Step program because we believe that it teaches a philosophy that is detrimental to healing and can lead to relapse." That is, Passages seeks to empower patients and heal their underlying conditions, rather than labeling them as addicts who have a disease. In this sense, its approach has elements of self-direction recommended by Farahany.

The therapists recognize four causes of addiction: (1) a chemical imbalance, (2) unresolved events from the past, (3) the inability to cope with current conditions, or (4) beliefs about their own health that are false. The first could require medical attention; the latter are more like mental health conditions (or, at least, conditions amenable to alternative therapies). In this regard, a few of the treatments that are offered include acupuncture, chemical dependency counseling, hypnotherapy, music therapy, and psychotherapy. Unlike 12-step programs, treatments are individualized and often involve one-on-one sessions with a treatment specialist.

The website states: "At Passages, we understand you are abusing drugs and alcohol to self-medicate underlying conditions in your life. To heal from chemical dependency-related issues, you will need to start by healing and treating the underlying conditions driving your addiction… The goal of treatment at Passages is to identify these underlying causes and address them in individual therapy so that they no longer lead to drug and alcohol use." In effect, the program seeks to encourage abusers to believe that someone is treating them, i.e., a whole person, rather than just treating a condition that is the same from one person to the next.

The universal tendency of humans to seek social contact can be put to good use here.[21] Study after study has reported that recovery programs that are supplemented by human contact did better than programs without social contact.

Both Marworth and Passages seek to recognize an individual's dignity, rather than requiring someone to acknowledge their fallen nature and be publicly "humble" about it. Bowen and collaborators (2013) reported that compared with treatment-as-usual (the control group), participants assigned to mindfulness-based relapse prevention and cognitive-behavioral relapse prevention treatment groups had significantly lower risk of relapse to substance use and heavy drinking, and among those who used substances, significantly fewer days of substance use and heavy drinking at a 6-month follow-up.

Toward the Future: From Rigid Abstinence to Harm Reduction

The following account of approaches to reducing drug addiction relies, in part, on Maia Szalavitz, *Undoing Drugs*.[22] Like Marworth and Passages, Szalavitz looks beyond older, rigid treatment modes. Thus, she embraces "harm reduction" movements that tried to reduce the harmful effects of the AIDS epidemic, i.e., *any positive change is to be valued.* For example, one of the ugly situations during that epidemic involved dirty needles: use them and die from an infection. Cleaning needles with bleach and supplying them to addicts saved lives.

---

[21] Pfaff DW. (2020) *Origins of Human Socialization*. Academic Press.

[22] Szalavitz M. (2022) *Undoing Drugs: How Harm Reduction is Changing the Future of Drug Addiction*. Balance.

Where does this story begin? (See Ref. 365, p. 44.) In 1986, Allan Parry attended a lecture on AIDS in Liverpool, U.K. The speaker was a public health expert from San Francisco who stated that (1) "effective prevention could not work without authorities genuinely partnering with affected communities," and (2) the best way to fight HIV was to provide clean needles. Parry immediately decided that Liverpool needed a syringe exchange program. The program expanded over the next several years. Then, he wondered about how to denominate the combination of needle exchange with "other compassionate approaches to drug users" (p. 49). The Liverpool group came up with the term "**harm reduction**." Simply trying to prevent young people from taking heroin had failed. Harm reduction "offered a new way to think about drugs" and focused more on "caring about the lives of people who use drugs." Undoing the policy focus on the drugs themselves allowed room to "rehumanize" policy. "The goal of a 'war on drugs' is simply stopping substance abuse" (p. 51); "the goal of harm reduction is making peoples' lives healthier and better." The effect of this shift was "a reconceptualization of the 'enemy' in drug policy." The idea was that "people who use drugs deserve the dignity, respect and right to self-determination" (p. 53), as with all humans. "Drug use is almost always a choice."

Szalavitz contends that addicts "could have behaved differently, or made better decisions." Thus, experts within the harm reduction movement contend that people addicted to drugs can exercise at least some degree of "free" choice (p. 54). For example, even though ostensibly addicted, the patient "may not be completely enslaved by drugs." The rigid 12-step programs, however, suggest that addicts are in a state of "complete powerlessness over drugs" and must therefore seek total abstinence. Szalavitz notes that if this were true, there would not have been such positive results from the syringe exchange and opioid maintenance. "Drugs did not turn people into robots or children," so "it was not acceptable to treat these fully equal human beings as though they were children or animals."

"Harm reductionists were meeting people where they're at" (p. 56). Their approach "offered tools and information drug users needed to reduce risk. Focusing on reducing harm can lead to better outcomes." That meant bleach education (to clean needles) and plastic bottles to take home methadone doses to try to "eliminate the risk of blood-borne disease entirely" (p. 62). As a result, "crime went down, health improved, and family lives were revitalized" (p. 65).

The new attitudes argued against the old American treatment system, where "the disease of addiction was progressive, anyone who continues to use drugs would always get worse" (p. 68). Szalavitz observes that "We [meaning Americans] value the lives of people who take these drugs less," and have the "stereotype of the addict as a lazy, devious, and violent sociopath" (p. 72). From the rigid abstinence point of view, anyone still using is not in recovery. "The result is that counselors must focus constantly on what is wrong, not what has improved" (p. 74).

Szalavitz states that the new, more flexible attitude is evident in the work of Jon Parker, trained at the Yale School of Public Health. "Needle exchange is necessary; bleach and teach is not enough." Parker took risks and "treated his clients respectfully," instructing them not to share any injecting equipment in a way that would spread infections. Such thinking aligns with the attitude of Stephen Joseph, NYC Health Commissioner, who cautions, "don't let the best be the enemy of the good." Demanding abstinence and criminalizing needle cleaning and exchange can kill people by exposing them to AIDS.

The Parker harm reduction approach "is now backed by research on numerous behaviors [see below] ranging from quitting smoking, treating eating disorders, increasing exercise to recycling." Parker states that "We're allowing people the means to stay AIDS-free" (p. 97). When he was a drug addict, Parker thought he had to completely change "from drug addict world to straight world." No! Gradual changes, for example, using needle exchanges (to ensure clean needles) and thus taking the first step of treatment "empowers the addict to realize he can make a difference in his own life." "He's doing something for his own self" (p. 98). "When they can make even a small difference in their life… they know they are doing something for the good of themselves and that's very powerful."

Parker's operative phrase, **"any positive change,"** provides the opportunity to make use of a basic technique in modern behavioral science. That is, the intellectual "father" of behaviorism, Harvard professor B.F. Skinner, working with animals learning experimental tasks, noticed that the experimenter could use variations in the topographical form of the behavioral response (e.g., paw vs. nose, beak vs. wing, running vs. swimming, left vs. right, up vs. down) or quantitative dimensions (e.g., intensity, duration, amplitude) of individual instances of the target behavior and *could selectively reinforce responses that are gradually more and more like the desired response form.*

Extending this line of thought eventually led to related concepts, such as "*successive approximations*" to the desired behavior, also called "response shaping." Regarding harm reduction, "any positive change" means that rather than requiring the patient to jump from addicted behavior to abstinence, even small gradual movements in the right direction can be rewarded. Step by step, the patient, exhibiting "successive approximations" to the desired behavior, can be eased into a drug-free life.

Saloner and collaborators report that harm reduction programs provide tools that enable drug users to use more safely, in a non-stigmatizing environment, without the goal of necessarily seeking treatment or abstinence.[23] Most harm reduction programs in the U.S. distribute sterile syringes and naloxone and safely dispose of used syringes and other drug-use supplies.

As a subject of human response-shaping, a young woman in San Francisco was addicted to cocaine. Her entire life was a mess. However, the "any positive change" counselor did NOT demand total abstinence. Instead, she took the first step of showing the woman how to manage her money. The addict had a small daughter, and they saw a beautiful dress in the window that was appropriate for her daughter but which she could not afford. Then, in a second step, "she realized that if she simply took two weekends off from crack, she could afford the coat." So, she took two weekends off (p. 127).

Many public-spirited urban workers think of safe housing as a basic human right (e.g., Lamberg).[24] According to Szalavitz, Keith Cylar, a social worker from Virginia, brought the principles of harm reduction to housing. The organization, Housing Works, exemplifies another aspect of a gradualist approach to improving addicts' lives (p. 122). It "pioneered housing for people with AIDS who used drugs" (p. 125). It initiated "scattered site" housing

---

[23] Saloner B, Heller D, Davis CS, & Sherman SG. (2025) Harm reduction: The neglected pillar of US drug policy. *Ann Rev Public Health* 46(1), 369–387.

[24] Lamberg C. (2018) *Neighborhood Success Stories: Creating and Sustaining Affordable Housing in New York*. Fordham Univ Press; Lamberg C. (2021) *Housing Security: A Section 8 Memoir.* Authors' Press

at first, meaning that AIDS patients were not all housed in the same building. "Eventually they owned several buildings" for housing such patients. "Harm reduction was the foundation for their work," superseding "standard rigid, infantilizing and punitive approaches." Cylar states that "if you can't keep people alive, you're never going to be able to help them into recovery." Housing Works also helped addicts manage their money from public assistance payments; Cylar's flexible approach dictated that after having helped an addict pay for essentials, they "chose to set aside a certain amount for crack" (p. 126), and "[t]he intention was not to be punitive or rigidly controlling."

Housing Works advocated a philosophy based on the idea that a person in an unstable situation on the street would be much less likely to get off drugs or alcohol. In New York, it began a program to provide modest housing for addicts, and "by 2010 the idea had become a principle of Federal housing policy" (p. 134).

Dan Bigg of the Chicago Recovery Alliance and John Szyler in Chicago came up with the crucial phrase: we're looking for "ANY POSITIVE CHANGE," where "positive" is defined by the patient. These examples could include getting a job, using a clean needle, going back to school, trying a new antidepressant, etc. (p. 147). At a meeting in Santa Cruz, both Dan and John started the Harm Reduction Working Group to formalize key ideas of harm reduction (p. 153–156). They wanted users to have "access to the tools to become healthy." Tacoma's Dave Purchase espoused "universal recognition of the inherent dignity in all life." That includes "supporting people where they are at, to make their own decisions, balancing the risks and benefits involved" (p. 159).

The University of Washington Addictive Behaviors Research Center's G. Alan Marlatt was famous for publishing research on harm reduction, with a special emphasis on brief interventions and relapse prevention.[25] For example, Logan and Marlatt wrote that harm reduction is an umbrella term for interventions aiming to reduce the problematic effects of certain behaviors. Although it was most frequently associated with addressing substance use, it is increasingly applied to other behavioral disorders. The article reviews the state of empirical research on harm reduction practices, including alcohol interventions for youth, college students, and a variety of other adult interventions. Marlatt also reviews nicotine replacement and opioid substitution, as well as needle exchanges and safe injection sites for intravenous drug users.

Dozens of peer-reviewed controlled trial publications provide support for the effectiveness of harm reduction for a multitude of clients and disorders without indications of unintended effects (for some examples, see below). Harm reduction interventions provide additional tools for clinicians working with clients who, for whatever reason, may not be ready, willing, or able to pursue full abstinence as a goal. Further, Marlatt put forward the concept of "urge surfing" as a coping mechanism for addiction. This strategy encourages the patient to view addictive urges as physical waves that rise in intensity, peak, and eventually crash and subside. The patient learns that urges, rather than building interminably until they become overwhelming, can subside rather quickly if they are not acted on.

Noyes and collaborators concentrated on adolescents and young adults (AYAs) who are highly vulnerable to substance use and substance use-related harms.[26] Existing harm reduction programs do not optimally serve AYAs, and there is insufficient data

---

[25] Logan DE & Marlatt GA. (2010) Harm reduction therapy: A practice-friendly review of research. *J Clin Psychol* 66(2), 201–214.

[26] Noyes E, Hausman E, Yeo EJ, *et al.* (2025) Harm reduction interventions for AYA who use opioids: A scoping review. *Drug Alcohol Depend* 272, 112677.

regarding harm reduction interventions specific to them, e.g., AYAs demonstrate different patterns of substance use and engagement with harm reduction compared to adults. However, they are open to harm reduction practices and informally engage in forms of harm reduction. A variety of harm reduction interventions are effective among AYAs, including naloxone training, fentanyl test strips, and safe injection facilities. They also respond well to programs that are convenient, private, and emphasize longitudinal relationship building with the community and providers. They may uniquely benefit from virtual programming, telehealth, and delivery services.

Jeziorska and collaborators reflect that Europe has been the first home for the harm reduction movement, acknowledging its values and principles relatively early, although not without challenges.[27] Built on successful experiences starting in the early 1980s, pioneering European countries committed to, invested in, and implemented a broad spectrum of harm reduction services over the years. The HIV/AIDS epidemic also helped to establish a broader recognition of the effectiveness of harm reduction policies in other countries as well. Pridgen and collaborators reviewed a wealth of research that demonstrated harm reduction interventions for substance use (SU) save lives and reduce risk for serious infectious diseases, such as HIV, hepatitis C, and other SU-related health conditions.[28] The U.S. has adopted several harm reduction interventions at the federal and state levels to combat SU-related harm. So, four 2025 reviews verify that "harm reduction is on the map."

---

[27] Jeziorska I, Martinelli TF, & Kools JP. (2025) 50 years of harm reduction in Europe: High time for transformation. *Harm Reduct J* 22(1), 94.

[28] Pridgen BE, Bontemps AP, Lloyd AR, *et al.* (2025) U.S. substance use harm reduction efforts: A review of the current state of policy, policy barriers, and recommendations. *Harm Reduct J* 22(1), 101.

Programs: ACTS UP and ADAPT

Two programs mentioned by Szailowitz deserve special attention. Abhiveer Singh in the Pfaff Lab describes ACTS UP (AIDS Coalition to Unleash Power) as a faith-based, volunteer-run program used in prisons and community churches. It works through lessons that come in weekly group courses; in each session, theory focuses on drug facts, object lessons, and personal testimony. The program focuses on positive reinforcement through spiritual identity, social belonging, and hope. It is used in some state correctional systems; its successes appear to be reported anecdotally. It also appears to be low-cost and would probably be ideal for participants who resonate with faith and storytelling.

ADAPT (Air Force Alcohol and Drug Abuse Prevention and Treatment) is the Air Force's in-house system for tackling alcohol and drug problems. It is set out in Air Force Instruction 44-121, and every base follows its playbook. First comes the prevention briefings for everyone. If someone starts slipping, they get a few motivational-style counseling sessions. If that is insufficient, they go into an eight-week outpatient class that teaches CBT (cognitive behavioral therapy) skills. After that, the staff keeps tabs on them for about a year. Really serious cases get sent to a civilian rehab center, but ADAPT still stays involved. This program uses two different arguments to get results from the participants. The first argument focuses on getting healthy and keeping one's career. The other argument is harsher — the emphasis on one losing their career if they keep on using drugs. Large-scale evaluations of ADAPT's brief-intervention and a random-breath-test package show that alcohol-related incidents fell 44% within six months among technical trainees and 16% across the four bases at a 12-month follow-up in a cluster-randomized trial.

Of the two programs, ACTS UP is faith-based; it tries to use positive reinforcement principles by replacing drug-related dopamine rewards with the natural rewards of hope, social connection, and purpose. On the other hand, ADAPT is primarily built on cognitive behavioral therapy and motivational interviewing, while adding structured skill-building with military accountability. It uses both intrinsic motivators (e.g., personal growth) and extrinsic motivators (e.g., career consequences) to lead to behavioral changes. So, while the ACTS UP program focuses more on change through community narrative and community values, ADAPT operates through evidence-based protocols. ADAPT is more structured and backed by official guidelines like Air Force Instruction 44-121, which lays out how the program works in different stages. ACTS UP does not have much formal research behind it, but it is used in prisons and community settings; it seems to work well because it leans into community, support, and personal stories.

Altruism

Dan Bigg states that "there's nothing more empowering than saving a life." He got addicted people to save each other.

Similarly, Pat Denning, in San Fran's Castro district, "brought harm reduction off the streets and into counseling sessions and rehabs." (p. 174) Bigg and Denning exhibit behavior that conforms to a basic law of human behavior, which states that humans behave altruistically.[29] In that book, we cite Michael Tomasello's work because he documents altruistic behavior in very young

---

[29] Pfaff DW & Sherman S. (2014) *The Altruistic Brain: How We are Naturally Good.* Oxford University Press, New York; Pfaff DW & Sherman S. (2025) *Laws of Human Behavior: Steps toward Hard Science.* The MIT Press, Cambridge.

children, who would not have received years of organized instructions about behavioral standards. In an example, one child needed help to get an out-of-reach object, and the second child got it for him. Similarly, young children showed more concern and prosocial behavior toward an adult who seemed to have been harmed. One of us (DP) drove to the Yale lab of Karen Wynn, whose experiments involved infants being shown little shows with puppets; in each show, there was a "good" puppet (helpful) and a "bad" puppet (mean, unhelpful). When presented with the two types of puppets after the show, the infants chose the "good" one significantly more frequently.

A large amount of data points to the PFC as being important for expressing altruistic behavior, though other cortical regions are also involved. We previously argued that altruistic acts can be considered as natural products of normal perceptual mechanisms — treating another person as how you would want others to treat you derives from underperforming perceptual pathways.

Problems and questions

Even as we appreciate the flexibility and individuality of the harm reduction approach to battling addiction, we must also wonder what happens when things go wrong with this approach. There is no "playbook." Should we trust in the skill of every therapist to react to setbacks optimally? How can we formulate a more generally applicable strategy? There are all too many ways for the addict to slip back into the habit. For example, the human behavioral law that "we reduce cognitive dissonance"[30] means that the recovering

---

[30] Pfaff DW & Sherman S. (2025) *Laws of Human Behavior: Steps toward Hard Science*. The MIT Press, Cambridge.

addict who slips up will take mental and behavioral steps to reduce the stress caused by the obvious discrepancy between his aspirations and his drug-taking behavior.

In the words of Mount Sinai's Eric Nestler, there is "a daunting challenge for neuroscientists: the requirement to characterize numerous neuronal and non-neuronal cell types in numerous limbic brain regions implicated in addiction and to refine those analyses to ensembles that are recruited by addictive drugs across the complex life cycle of addiction."[31] Meeting this challenge will take time, both in the basic research laboratory and in the clinic.

Next research steps: The neurobiology of emotion

Underlying all the neurobiology referred to in this book is the question of emotion. How does the addict feel from day to day? Would harm reduction steps make him or her feel better? From a neurobiological research point of view, we might see the development of opportunities to study the mechanisms underlying emotions to help in the job of harm reduction, since all forms of drug addiction manifestly have very strong emotional content.

For decades, neuroscientists have known that the neurons most important for the performance of emotion-bearing behaviors could be found in the ancient forebrain — not the cerebral cortex on top of the brain but near the bottom of the forebrain in structures called the amygdala, the preoptic area, the hypothalamus, and the bed nucleus of the stria terminalis. These neurons can be drawn into the explanation of simple emotional responses, for example, sex, fear, and aggression. These are mechanisms that work instantaneously.

---

[31] Nestler E. (2025) The biology of addiction. *Sci Signal* 18(872), eadq0031.

More recently, a few scientists have begun to ask how it is that some emotions may persist for a long while. Yes, the immediate response to an emotion-inducing stimulus can easily be found in the activities of neurons in specific places in the brain, but what about emotional states that last a long time, e.g., grief? Scientists at Stanford have recently used novel computational techniques to follow electroencephalographic activity, long-lasting brain-wide waves that can be disrupted with a drug like ketamine, which can also disrupt emotional experiences (in humans).[32] This work represents one recent step forward in the analyses of emotional mechanisms in the brain, which hopefully will find applications in the continuing work to deal with drug addiction.

Reflection

Writing *Drugs of Abuse* required some heavy lifting, for example, in examining the effects of some drugs on various brain mechanisms. But we anticipated this. We did not anticipate much of the enjoyment in writing it. Who would have imagined, when setting out to write about addictive drugs, that they would be examining the labels on King Tut's wine jars, or laughing with an 18th-century dramatist at the pretentiousness of snuff-taking? While addiction is dead serious, its origins in more innocent pleasures were a bit of comic relief (albeit a cold comfort).

We first conceived this book to provide information that now appears in Section 2, so that readers could understand the neurochemistry of addictive drugs. How do these drugs work in the

[32] Kauvar I, Richman EB, Liu TX, *et al.* (2025) Conserved brain-wide emergence of emotional response from sensory experience in humans and mice. *Science* 20(XX), eadt3971.

brain and become so addictive? Why, ultimately, is it so hard to quit? But as we wrote, we recognized that these questions bear on serious moral issues: for example, the amount of agency that humans have in getting "hooked" — is it all just chemical, or can willpower overcome the powerful mechanism that makes addiction possible? As we began thinking about these questions, we realized that we had to delve deeper, which is how *Drugs of Abuse* began to take its present shape.

The most difficult part of this book to write was the last, concerning present and still-evolving initiatives to combat addiction. The subject is a moving target: recovery is so challenging, and attitudes toward it are changing. Some serious professionals are moving on from 12-step programs that demand total abstinence, embracing flexible harm-reduction models that seek any positive change and recognize addicts' individual needs. Additionally, prospective high-tech approaches will likely include transcranial magnetic stimulation, deep-brain micro-stimulation, and localized neuron-specific chemical manipulation. We report these developments in real-time.

Index

www.ingramcontent.com/pod-product-compliance
Lightning Source LLC
La Vergne TN
LVHW051051210926
848486LV00002B/74

* 9 7 8 9 8 1 9 8 3 1 4 7 0 *